DR WOLFGANG LUTZ AND HIS CHICKENS

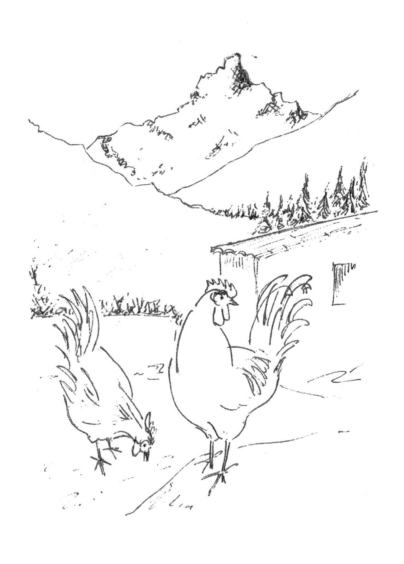

Dr Wolfgang Lutz and his Chickens:

Carbohydrate and Arterial Health

Valerie Bracken

JUST PERHAPS?

EDINBURGH

Also by Valerie Bracken
Uncle Wolfi's Secret: A Tribute to Dr Wolfgang Lutz
My Life Without Bread: Dr Lutz at 90

First published in Great Britain in 2019 by
JUST PERHAPS?

www.justperhaps.co.uk

ISBN: 9781703547726

The purpose of this book is to educate and inform. It is sold with the understanding that the publisher and author shall have neither liability nor responsibility for any injury caused or alleged to be caused by the information or ideas contained in this book, the contents of which should not be construed as medical advice. Each person's health needs are unique. To obtain guidance appropriate for your situation, please consult your doctor.

A catalogue record for this book is available from the British Library

This book is dedicated to Dr Wolfgang Lutz
1913 – 2010
to whom I will always be grateful,
with my thanks to Sarah and Mark

JUST PERHAPS?

aims to celebrate the work of pioneering doctors
who have dedicated their lives to an aspect of medical
practice that lies outside the mainstream yet
which – just perhaps – has something of
vital importance to offer us.

CONTENTS

FOREWORD

Dr Wolfgang Lutz pioneered low carbohydrate
nutrition from the late 1950s and spent half a
century using it with his patients and observing its
efficacy. It was my privilege, over the last 15 years
of his life, to intermittently assist Dr Lutz with
presenting his work in the English language. The
following is taken from a large unpublished work
that had been in preparation for and with Dr Lutz,
hence the use of the first person in the narrative.
The draft was written at the turn of the century and
Dr Lutz personally approved the script, which was
later summarised in my book *My Life without
Bread: Dr Lutz at 90*. Recent interest in the results
of his chicken investigations has encouraged me to
put this manuscript into the public domain.

Valerie Bracken

Please note that no part of this book is to be construed as
medical advice.

1 ALLAYING FEARS

Cholesterol and animal fats

Over recent years, concern for the supposedly harmful role of animal fats, and particularly of cholesterol, has left many other aspects of health in the shade. I expressed my views on the significance of cholesterol and blood fats in several books. As early as 1970, I wrote that these were not of such significance for practical medicine that one had to know their blood level in every circumstance. My views on this have not changed. Of all the blood chemistry levels that I took in patients who came to see me, it was the cholesterol level that caused me the least concern – or rather, that would have interested me the least if the patient, as if mesmerised, were not already anxiously waiting to know his or her cholesterol reading.

Once officialdom, too, had taken it upon itself to care for the cholesterol level of its people, I felt duty-bound to present a summary of the cholesterol problem myself. Therefore, in 1988, I attempted a new evaluation of the question in a book entitled: *Cholesterin und tierische Fette* (cholesterol and animal fats). Over to Prof. Glatzel who wrote the foreword:

> In this situation, Prof. Lutz was one of the first to point out clearly that cholesterol not only was a component of many foodstuffs that had been eaten for thousands of years, but that it was also an integrating constituent of the human body.
>
> He was one of the few who showed in a well-informed and factual way that many of the studies, which had been undertaken world-wide, left a host of open questions. Not all experiences can be reduced to a common denominator. Too much cholesterol may be harmful - but how much is too much!

Do cholesterol-lowering medications really achieve clinically the results that many hope for from them? And at what level does the cholesterol level of the "normal" healthy person lie? Question after question - and a few more ought to be added here: does it make sense for our Minister for Research and Science to spend millions on the cholesterol level of German citizens? Does it do any good to do without cholesterol-containing egg yolks, even though they cause hardly any rise in the serum cholesterol? Could it be possible that the rise in serum cholesterol during stress situations is an important process of adaptation?

In short, there are still enough open questions on the theme of cholesterol for one to want to listen with interest to what Dr Lutz has to say.

Foreword by Prof. Hans Glatzel (in Lutz, 1988)

It was good of Prof. Glatzel to say this last, but I wonder how many people have actually listened and how many have really thought about it. That foreword was written in the 1980s and it seems to me that there are still just as many open questions as there were then. In the meantime, too many scientists have identified with the 'fat theory' (i.e. that cholesterol and animal fats are responsible for heart problems, arteriosclerosis and so on) for one to expect a rapid reversal of its influence. I once wrote that the saying of Max Planck applies here, namely that a new scientific truth is not achieved by way of convincing its opponents who then declare themselves converted, but rather by its opponents gradually dying out and by the new generation being already familiarised with the truth.

I was then already 75 and had been living quasi as early man for about thirty years. I was hoping to experience a change of trend in the field of human nutrition during my lifetime.

Most unfortunately, the fat theory has continued to dominate the teaching of nutrition.

My fear is that the new generation, far from being 'familiarised with the truth', is growing up accepting as true the false tenets of the fat theory and so choosing their food accordingly. Perhaps it will take another generation yet before the situation is seen for what it is, namely that: 'the public is being deceived by the greatest health scam of the [twentieth] century' (Mann 1993). Let us hope the twenty-first century will tell a different tale.

To get to the truth of the matter, Prof. G. V. Mann of Vanderbilt University, Nashville had set up a forum, aptly named the Veritas Society. The resultant report, from which the above quote is taken, sums up the evaluation by scientists and was published in 1993 as: *Coronary Heart Disease: The dietary sense and nonsense*. Earlier, Mann had written his sensational article: Diet heart, end of an era (1967). There were others too who opposed the widely held interpretation of the big American field studies.

Dissenting voices include that of Prof. Glatzel himself (1974, 1982), who later worked at the Max Planck Institute for Nutritional Physiology at Dortmund. My compatriot Prof. Hans Kaunitz (1976, 1978), of Columbia University, New York, has been fighting for years against the idea that dietary fat, and especially animal fat, is at all implicated in the development of arteriosclerosis. It was from Kaunitz that the repair theory originated : the idea that, in the first instance, cholesterol is deposited in places where repairs are needed. It is a theory I favour myself and to which I will return.

The work Towards healthful Diets was written in 1980 for the US Academy of Science by Prof. Robert Olson, then of the University of St. Louis. After thorough perusal of the literature, he concluded that Americans should not deviate from their previous lifestyle since the available scientific data did not support the recommendation to avoid foodstuffs containing cholesterol and animal fats.

This sentiment was echoed by Oliver (1983) who, to introduce his own plea that blanket measures to prevent heart disease should be dropped on the grounds of lack of evidence of any general benefit to the community, calls on Oliver Cromwell's dramatic plea:

> I beseech you, in the bowels of Christ, think it possible that you might be mistaken.

Amongst others who have spoken out in similar vein are Reaven (1976), Ahrens junior (1976), McMichael (1977) and Groves (2000).

Practising physicians, too, have stressed the importance of keeping traditional fats in the diet: among these are Doctors Atkins (1972), Cleave (1974) and Kwasniewski (1999). A short and very readable summary of the situation is given by retired Scottish general practitioner, Dr Walter Yellowlees, in his chapter on fats in his book: *Doctor in the Wilderness* (1993). As you see, I am not quite alone in opposing the condemnation of cholesterol and animal fats.

For those readers impatient to know more details of the intrigue, the misleading epidemiology, the commercial pressures, the inaccurate reportage of study findings and biased selection of study material, the short-term and one-sided experiments and other ingredients that went into creating the false dogma concerning animal fat, they could do no better than to read from cover to cover Prof. Mann's book, quoted above; it is a splendid evaluation of the whole scenario.

Medical opinion of Western Europe is, however, largely dominated by the (sometimes fictitious) results of American research and American influence still holds sway. And:

> After all, no one likes to be told that the notions upon which he may have built and promoted his career have turned out to be wrong. (Lewin 1988)

So this business is not nearly at an end: the trend is for the proportion of fat in our food (the mythical average intake) to be further reduced and to be replaced by yet more carbohydrates.

What are we to make of it all? A few eminent scientists and physicians condemn the fat theory and many eminent scientists and physicians uphold it and advise government and nutritional bodies to ensure the populace complies with their advice. I had long ago cast my own vote by advocating a diet that permitted my patients to eat as much animal fat and protein as they liked.

Meanwhile, meat and animal fats are disappearing from the shelves of supermarkets in favour of packet cereals, bread and bakery goods, rice and potatoes, vegetables and fruit. It is hardly surprising that we are seeing slim figures give way to the broad hips and paunches that are now so commonplace amongst us. In some places it is hardly possible to get hold of good, natural fats any more. I love fat and feel that really good cooking cannot be achieved without it. But when I ask for fat pork to cook, the butcher just shrugs his shoulders and says that the fat had already been taken off before he got the meat!

The vital role of cholesterol in our bodies

Let us stay for a moment with the contentious subject of cholesterol. For what is often overlooked is that cholesterol is part of the make-up of our body which, far from being a villain of the piece, is in fact absolutely vital to us – so much so that we could not live without it.

As our body's major transport system, the bloodstream carries in its flow a lot of the materials that are needed in various places of the body, the blood taking the wherewithal to the cells for them to make energy and to do all their other tasks, including rebuilding themselves. As one of the building blocks of the body, cholesterol is just such a material and the bloodstream carries it round the body to and from the cells as required. This is a normal bodily procedure, so healthy blood will have a fluctuating amount of cholesterol present.

Cholesterol is present not only in the blood but throughout our body. It is one of our essential structural materials. Along with phospholipids, it helps to build and maintain the integrity of the walls of the trillions of cells in our body. It is also abundant in the grey matter of our nervous tissue including the brain, as well as in our adrenal glands and ovaries, and it is what our steroid hormones are made from. Having many functions, it is needed in all tissues and in every cell of the body.

Where does this much needed and seemingly ubiquitous substance come from? Well, some of it may come from the fat we eat. The body can use the cholesterol it derives from fatty food fairly directly: the handling of cholesterol is fairly simple since the cholesterol that is eaten during our meals is chemically similar to the cholesterol that occurs in our body tissues, any excess being excreted in the bile.

But just because cholesterol is both a constituent of food and of our bodies, this does not mean that the two should be equated. Even if it remains a similar substance and does not need to be processed to the extent of some other substances, the body can still choose whether or not to reuse the cholesterol as well as in which location and for what purpose. The workings of the body are complex yet discriminating.

Moreover, since cholesterol is vital to our well-being and since our body puts our interests first, there is a fallback position lest dietary fat may be in short supply: namely our body has the ability to manufacture its own cholesterol from the protein and carbohydrate that we eat. Given the present zeal for eating so little fat, it is well for us, I think, that nature has provided these failsafe arrangements!

All internal body substances that are essential to life are necessarily 'good' in the sense of being beneficial – a truism that we do not always bear in mind. Yet, though beneficial at their intended internal concentrations, by their very nature all vital substances may be harmful and even fatal when present in amounts outside this range. These days the focus of attention is on having 'too much' cholesterol, even if how much is too much is still an open question. But, given how essential it is for our health, might not the question of 'too little' cholesterol be of vital importance and need to be addressed?

Surely then, cholesterol cannot be as 'bad' as it is made out to be! Are we sure that we should be trying so hard to get rid of it from our bodies or that it is safe to eat medicated foods targeted to that end? Should we not rather question the wisdom of advocating the indiscriminate reduction of cholesterol?

The importance of arterial health

It is said that a man is as old as his arteries. Now, arteries are central to our body's economy, since they carry our oxygenated 'life blood' to the whole body: tissues, limbs, internal organs and brain. Since arteries are carriers of the blood, which is being pumped forcibly along them by the heart, they need to be thick and strong and yet giving: thick and strong to withstand the pulsation without damage and yet with enough 'give' or elasticity to accommodate it. Since arteries are vital, they need to be protected and they also need to facilitate the smooth flowing of blood.

Hence the artery wall is provided with three layers or coats. There is a protective outer fibrous layer, composed of connective tissue, which is called the tunica adventitia. There is a strong middle coat, which is muscular and elastic, called the tunica media, which is much the thickest layer. The innermost coat, the tunica intima, is composed of yellow elastic tissue, on the inner surface of which there is a layer of plate-like so-called endothelial cells, which are smooth and flat and form the lining of the blood vessel. This smooth inner lining surrounds the space in the middle – the hollow where the blood flows, called the lumen.

In the body, there is a whole 'tree' of arteries, branching from the main trunk, the aorta, which receives blood straight from the heart, into smaller arteries, into still smaller ones called arterioles, and thence to the tiny capillaries where the exchange of gases, foodstuffs and waste takes place. The aorta, the largest blood vessel, is nearest the pump and so, since it receives the full force of the impetus from the heart to start the blood on its journey round the body, it needs to be very distensible. Consequently, it has less muscle but far more elastic fibres than the smaller arteries. In the abdomen, the aorta bifurcates into the iliac arteries which continue to the femoral arteries of the legs. This fork is subject to more mechanical stress than other parts of the aorta from the pulsation of the blood.

The words systole and diastole crop up when a doctor does a blood pressure reading. These elastic fibres distend in systole, i.e. when the heart contracts, forcing the blood into the aorta (which is when the blood pressure is greatest) and recoil in diastole, i.e. the lull in between before the next contraction of the heart. As this alternating dilation and recoil of the arteries is a vital adjunct to the work of the heart, you can see why any stiffening and loss of elasticity in their walls will have important consequences for health.

Hardening of the arteries

Arteriosclerosis is a degenerative condition of the arterial blood vessels, popularly known as hardening of the arteries. This is because, in one form of arteriosclerosis, the walls of the arteries do in fact thicken, harden and lose their elasticity. This process may or may not give rise to symptoms, depending on which arteries are affected. Those most commonly involved are the aorta, the coronary, cerebral, iliac and femoral arteries. In other words, it is most likely to be a problem for the heart, the brain, the hips and legs.

The hardening of the arteries in old age often entails a rigidity of the middle coat of the blood vessel and there are many stages of the process, including the deposition of connective tissue, fats and calcium salts. Because of the latter, the condition is also called chalking or furring of the arteries, as the arteries 'fur up' a bit like water pipes do in hard water areas. In extreme cases, these deposits of lime may change the arteries into brittle calcareous tubes, very liable to tearing from slight injuries. This type of hardening is usually confined to older people, when it may be accompanied by high blood pressure, diabetes, gout or chronic kidney disease, but not necessarily so.

However, the process of arteriosclerosis can begin very early in life. Patchy thickening of the arterial walls is known to occur even in the newborn, especially where the arteries divide (Stehbens in Mann 1993). Milk spots, where lipids are being integrated into the inner wall of the blood vessel, can often already be seen in the arteries of children. This form of degenerative change is strictly termed atherosclerosis, though the two terms are often used interchangeably, as I do myself.

It was with this latter type of arteriosclerosis, rather than the brittle type, that I was particularly concerned. The patchy thickening of the inner wall is accompanied by the deposition of fatty material containing a high proportion of cholesterol and other lipids, but can contain a number of other substances such as smooth muscle cells and fibrous tissue, which William Stehbens refers to as: 'the accumulation of lipid-rich debris in the thickened intima'.

Atherosclerosis, in other words, is characterised by fatty streaks, known as striae, and lumpy bits on the inside of the artery walls; these lumpy bits are known as plaques and can be made of a cholesterol-containing yellowish material. (This used to be called atheroma, from the Greek for porridge.) You will see the resemblance, at least to badly made porridge, in the photograph in chapter 3.

Just as we cannot afford a loss of elasticity in our arteries, nor can we afford our 'tubes' to get too narrow. This, unfortunately, is another thing that tends to happen in arteriosclerosis: the deposits in the inner walls tend to get bigger with time and, as the plaques enlarge and the intima itself increases in thickness, the lumen of the artery becomes smaller and smaller.

In due course, the lumen may be so narrowed that the blood flow is obstructed and becomes easily blocked, thus predisposing to a clot or thrombosis; or else a clot may form round a plaque and then get detached into the bloodstream and block a narrower artery. Either way, if this blocking occurs in the coronary arteries that supply the heart muscle, the heart is deprived of the oxygen it needs to function: the result is all too often the greatly feared coronary thrombosis.

This is the sudden death at the rostrum or steering wheel at the prime of life. If it occurs in the arteries of the legs, it may cause gangrene, if in the brain, a stroke. Arteriosclerosis may or may not lead to such dire consequences, but it is this sudden and very dramatic outcome of a slow, insidious and gradually progressive disease of the arteries, which has led this condition to be in the spotlight of international interest and research.

The task before me

It was quite early on that diet was put under this spotlight. I have been darting about in time but in terms of what I have to tell, we are now in the late 1950s/early 1960s. At that time, arteriosclerosis had long been considered a precursor of heart attacks and strokes. But now, the idea was gaining ground that arteriosclerosis is caused by eating saturated fat, and especially by eating cholesterol.

This was where I came in, for both these substances are found in all animal food, the latter being especially plentiful in food such as egg yolks, butter and liver – in fact, in the sort of food I was recommending. The worry, which I alluded to at the beginning of chapter one ran something like this:

> "I feel fine now on your diet, Dr Lutz, but am I storing up trouble for the future? Will this diet cure my present troubles but, unbeknown to me, gradually build up problems in my arteries because of its fat content?"

It was a fair question, for what was easier to imagine than that my diet would raise the cholesterol level in the blood, the cholesterol then attaching itself to the arterial walls with the alarming consequences already mentioned.

Here I must stress that the presence of arteriosclerosis does not mean one will necessarily have a heart attack or stroke, for these can occur when arteriosclerosis is only slight and yet, in people with severe arteriosclerosis, thrombotic complications may be completely absent. Nevertheless, even if heart attacks and strokes do not always follow, arteriosclerosis is seen as a big so-called risk factor – a likely antecedent to such misfortunes.

I was not anxious for myself on this score but I obviously wanted to allay any fears or uneasiness amongst my many patients as to the possibility of long-term deleterious effects. To do this, I wanted to find a practical way of demonstrating to them that the development of arteriosclerosis was unlikely on my diet or, at the very least, any tendency towards it would not be aggravated and that my diet was more likely to promote the health of their arteries than the reverse.

The task before me was two-fold: to reassure my patients and to demonstrate that the fat theory was based on a false premise. For this task, I needed concrete evidence that animal fats were not at the bottom of the modern scourge of heart attacks and strokes. Moreover, there was a pressing need to show that carbohydrates probably were.

2 CHICKEN FEED

Looking for evidence

My task was now to look for evidence – evidence moreover that was demonstrable and replicable – to show that the general beneficial effect of my diet extended to the health of the arteries and that it was likely to give protection against arteriosclerosis. It was one of my personal guidelines for evaluating diets that any diet worth following should not swap one disease for another. Obviously, I would not knowingly put my own patients at risk.

But how could I show that I was not already doing so? Somehow, I had to find a way of demonstrating that my way was a safer way than that which my patients had been used to. This was especially necessary given the way arteriosclerosis develops so slowly and gives so few warning signs. If I were wrong in my proposed diet, it could be years before I found out the serious cost to patients of my error.

Arteriosclerotic change seems usually to begin with some sort of damage or injury to the inner layer of the arterial blood vessels, most frequently to the aorta; the reasons for these so-called lesions (or damage) are still much disputed, one being mechanical stress. But there is, I feel, another reason over and above possible mechanical stress – and one that is particularly pertinent to any consideration of carbohydrate in relation to the health of the arteries – and that is the catabolic overload consequent on the overproduction of adrenal hormones (cortisol and thyroid T_3 and T_4) engendered by the extra gluconeogenesis needed because of the disorder brought about by the overconsumption of dietary carbohydrates.

Let me explain. Put simply, anabolic processes are about building up and catabolic ones about breaking down. Both are absolutely essential and complementary body processes, only harmful when out of balance, especially for prolonged periods.

To function, the body needs fuel. Whereas anabolic activity involves the use of energy to create matter, providing fuel is a catabolic process, that is it involves the breakdown of matter to create energy. We need fuel night and day, awake or asleep, to power what goes on in our body. Nature has given us a beautifully intricate system of energy provision to ensure that this need is covered all the time.

As a distinct species we, today, are of the genus Homo sapiens. For something like 150,000 years Homo sapiens was nomadic. Living as hunter/gatherers, the availability of food was of necessity sporadic: sometimes short, sometimes plentiful, often sparse. Yet, to stay alive, hearts must beat continually and, for survival, the energy to hunt without eating must be maintained sometimes over days at a time.

Nature in her wisdom, as she did with other higher animals, chose the most energy-efficient fuel for our own internal use: namely fat. How could it be otherwise? Our energy producers, the cell mitochondria, do use protein and carbohydrate as well as fat to make energy but mainly fat, and this energy is on tap as needed. And, to cater for the necessarily unreliability of an intermittent food supply, nature did not tie energy provision to the last meal or even to mealtimes generally.

Our inherent design therefore is to use fat as our primary source of internal fuel, with protein and carbohydrate as secondary sources. Fat is not only an energy-efficient source, but is readily available either from food or from the fat cells where it is stored and from where, in a state of health, it can be deposited and accessed in micro-seconds. Apart from a small amount of sugar that can be assimilated straight from the mouth, fat has its own much quicker route to being used than most foodstuff since it does not first need to go through the whole digestive process when eaten.

There is a small amount of carbohydrate present in animal food and this our system was used to. In the days of our Ice-Age brethren, our hormonal system would therefore have been well balanced with the individual hormones co-operating harmoniously and our energy supply would be constant and independent of mealtimes.

The hormone insulin has many functions and is routinely secreted after a meal: the amount of insulin rising a little and then as naturally subsiding without making any extra demands on the other hormones involved. And, so it would have been whilst living almost entirely on animal food – or more recently say, with the Inuit still living on their ancient diet.

However, within the last 10,000 years or so, cereals gradually enter the picture and, with the introduction of grain, settled farming and the chance to grow and store food. This was a turning point in our history for it marked not only the end of pre-history and the decline of what we choose to call primitive man but, for good or ill, it ushered in the beginnings of what we call civilisation. I say for good or ill as, although there were undoubted benefits in terms of inventiveness and creativity, it also ushered in many health problems including dental caries – and cancer?

Tooth decay is an example of catabolic imbalance, where the breaking down predominates over defence and self-repair. One reason for this might well be that this new foodstuff had more carbohydrate content than formerly expected by our bodies, another that grain itself is suspect in this regard.

Populations increased and, even today, the part played by the ingestion of grain say, on the stimulation of sex hormones is not sufficiently recognised nor the infertility that can follow prolonged stimulation. Over time, our intake of carbohydrate gradually increased both from grain and other sources.

One compromise too far?

For us the question is this: with the increase of plant food in our diet, how did our bodies cope with more carbohydrate? What were the hormonal mechanisms by which our bodies managed this change? This is, I think, important to understand.

Naturally, our bodies did their best to adapt to the new situation. Here I do not mean they adapted in the sense of the biological adaptation of our genes: it was rather that our bodies made adjustments, they 'made do', as it were. And, naturally too, there were costs and consequences to this.

In terms of nutrition, meat with its fat (in the sense of animal food generally) is the original and best food for human beings. Together with water, it constitutes a complete food and will sustain excellent health, whereas grain alone does not and cannot. The protein in grain is incomplete and needs to be supplemented, and it contains certain chemicals which inhibit the absorption of certain elements necessary for health.

This is one cost of reliance on cereal. Another is that since grain is nutritionally inferior to meat, those people who first took up cereal eating with enthusiasm, were smaller in stature and a little less strong. This is well documented by Palaeontologists.

One consequence of this transition to a foodstuff containing more carbohydrate than formerly, was that this inevitably meant new demands were made on our regulatory systems. A new stress – a new challenge if you like – is a new stimulus to the body which demands a response. Some of this response is managed by our hormonal system.

In terms of our basic metabolism, when we eat carbohydrate, whether in the form of sugar or starch, it is converted by the body into sugar. This enters the bloodstream and, since there is only so much sugar that can be tolerated in the bloodstream, not just insulin but our entire hormonal system is called on to make appropriate adjustments.

Yes, it is the special job of insulin to keep this sugar within safe bounds, but it is helped by a team of hormones that I often refer to as the sugar squad, of which insulin is the leader. When the sugar level is considered too high i.e. more than would have been expected on our ancient diet, this squad is mobilised: extra insulin is secreted. This hormone sees to the removal of the extra sugar from the blood, which is either put immediately into use for the production of energy, converted into glycogen (the only way sugar can be stored i.e. as animal starch stored in the liver and muscles for emergency use) or converted into fat for future use and for which there is plenty of storage capacity. So far so good, you say.

As eating more carbohydrate became a habitual part of our daily diet, we developed a sort of compromise between what we might think of as the old way and the new way. A middling amount of carbohydrate say, is eaten with a meal; in order that priority is given to lowering the sugar level, insulin secretion immediately rises to meet the need as does that of the rest of the squad, except the level growth hormone which falls.

In this way, insulin rules the hormonal roost straight after eating. Then, after about two hours, the situation reverts to what the body considers as normal, the level of growth hormone rises and fat is again used as the main fuel, as it continues to be so used overnight.

Thus our original metabolic pattern, which has been with us for 150,000 years or so (and very much longer if we count our predecessors), developed over the last few thousand years one could say, a compromise system of 'half and half', which alternated between fat and sugar being used as its main fuel. Though it was not a recipe for excellent health, it has come to be viewed as standard hormonal behaviour. It elicited and still elicits many health problems, yet for some people it still works reasonably well. So far, not quite so good.

However, if a much higher level of carbohydrate is eaten and if this level of carbohydrate continues regularly over a period of time, then it is definitely over-consumption and the situation changes yet again. This is especially so if, as is seen frequently these days, there are sugary or starchy snacks between meals as well as at bedtime. By continually giving priority to the removal of unwanted sugar, the body now gets into the self-protective habit of using sugar as its primary fuel, with fat and protein secondary and with the use of both fat and protein partially blocked by insulin to allow this self-defence.

Surely, you say, once supper has been dealt with, there is still all night to use fat for fuel. I think not. My own feeling is that, once this habit of sugar use settles in, a mere eight hours before that morning cup of tea with two spoons of sugar, is insufficient to reconvert to fat as the main fuel source.

In this scenario, we have a situation in which the body is forced to run – and almost continually – predominantly on a fuel which is only half as efficient as that more suited to its metabolic design, which disturbs its system of hormonal regulation and which brings serious consequences in its wake.

In this way, in only half a century, misled by the fat theory into reducing fat in the diet and backed by official commendation of carbohydrate as the natural basis for our food intake, for many people man's original pattern of fuel use has been turned completely upside down.

Does this matter? Yes, it certainly does and for many reasons. One is that, on this new program and with the supply of sugar on an as-needed basis curtailed for technical reasons to do with the production of energy (see Allan & Lutz 2000), there will now not be enough sugar either in the bloodstream or from the meagre stores of glycogen in the liver and muscles to supply this sugar overnight. To do this, led by the adrenal hormones (cortisol and thyroid T_3 and T_4), protein is therefore scavenged from the body to make into sugar. I have been known to call this the 'nightly protein sacrifice of the carbohydrate-eater'.

This is the gluconeogenesis mentioned earlier: namely the conversion of protein into sugar, including body protein. Gluconeogenesis is a lifesaver in starvation and a wholesome process when it is a matter of recycling body waste such as worn-out cells that are being replaced. But it is unwholesome and damaging when, for instance, it means robbing our arteries of protein from their inner protein-laden walls. In fact, this slow erosion of the artery walls is thought to be one of the initiating factors in arteriosclerosis, with fatty deposits secondary: these being put there by the body to repair this damage by plugging the holes with fat.

In this regard, with insulin raised to sort out the excess sugar and the raised catabolic hormones slowly eroding our tissues, there is another reason why it matters and that is the simultaneous lowering of the growth hormone. The growth hormone is in charge not just of growth in the young but of the constant repair and renewal of our tissues during the whole of our life: a habitually low level of growth hormone means not only less resistance to infection (the growth hormone being closely connected to the immune system), but also constantly poorer tissue quality and poor repairs, including to the arteries.

Moreover, the effort of constant adjustment by our hormones can lead to their exhaustion and eventual breakdown.

Could it be that over the last 50 years or so, our new habit of overwhelming the body with too many sugars and starches has forced the body into one compromise too far? Could it be that in this manner we have unwittingly brought many of these chronic degenerative conditions on ourselves by our choice of food? Sadly, one only has to look at the health statistics of affluent countries for an answer!

Be that as it may, my immediate questions are these: might it be possible to show that, on the right diet, all this damaging hormonal activity would not happen in the first place? On a diet that corresponded to nature's requirements for us, less unwanted substances would be in the bloodstream to start with and surely we would, in any case, be far healthier and so our body tissues, including the walls of our arteries, would be stronger and constant repair therefore less necessary?

At best, in terms of our arteries, there would then be no underlying weakness that eventually gave rise to arteriosclerosis. Even if all that could be achieved by dietary means was a lessening and a slowing down of arterial degeneration, then my hope was that its later complications such as thinning of the middle layer, tearing and ulceration of the intima, ischaemia, thrombosis, rupture and haemorrhage might be avoided.

I was therefore not without optimism. As you may imagine, I was keen to get on with my investigations straight away. It would take too many years to sit around and patiently await its absence in my patients, which is precisely what I would hope to see on my diet – nothing but healthy arteries and a lack of the development of arteriosclerosis. Nor, for reasons already given, could I wait for the consensus of medical opinion to come to my rescue. The only way forward was to instigate my own research.

It was with all this in mind that I considered animal-feeding experiments. Thus it was that, very early on in my 'low carbohydrate' days, I embarked on an interesting series of feeding trials, which took nearly ten years to complete. My main object was to try and ascertain whether the amount of carbohydrate (and incidentally of fat) eaten in the food bore any definite relationship to the incidence of arterial disease.

Why I chose chickens

In the past, many experiments to do with arteriosclerosis have been carried out on purely herbivorous animals in the hope of learning something about our own illnesses. I hardly need to point out that to eat animal protein and fat is unnatural for herbivores, whose body systems are therefore not geared to receive it: comparisons are consequently fraught with difficulty and the results not surprisingly inconclusive or even misleading.

Take wild rabbits. When rabbits, which are herbivores, are given food containing fat and cholesterol, such unnatural feeding causes great problems and they react adversely. Yes, lesions occur in their arteries but, importantly, the lesions produced are very different from those occurring in humans and for different reasons.

Rabbits need cholesterol for the functioning of their bodies just as much as we do. However, there is a fundamental difference between rabbits and ourselves. Whereas our own bodies expect to receive cholesterol from food but have internal provision to manufacture our own if necessary, say in hard times, the bodies of rabbits do not anticipate getting cholesterol from their food and here lies the rub. As rabbits manufacture all the cholesterol they need inside their own bodies, nature has not equipped them with a feedback mechanism to switch off their own intrinsic cholesterol production in the event of receiving unexpected cholesterol from outside (Enig, in Mann 1993).

Blood vessels are of similar construction in all higher animals yet, as we have seen, not all animals develop arteriosclerosis in the way humans do. So it does matter which animal you choose to compare with humans! Take apes: apes despite having a common ancestry and also sharing a lot of genetic material with us, exhibit a variable tissue response to dietary fats, both between and amongst species. For these reasons, I discounted both rabbits and apes, which in those days usually served as the usual experimental animals for studying the development of arteriosclerosis.

To gain understanding that would be of practical use, I felt it necessary to look for detailed similarities between humans and the trial animal in three respects:

31

a) histologically, i.e. similarity in tissue reaction
b) biochemically, i.e. similarity in the chemical composition of the fats that are laid down in the artery walls
c) nutritionally, i.e. similarity in their basic diet – their original type of diet before the intervention of man.

I therefore thought about choosing chickens. Hens, I know, stand a long way from humans on the evolutionary chain but it seems that they suffer nevertheless from a similar type of arteriosclerosis to that which occurs in humans. This I had learned from an article on atherosclerosis in hens, written in 1956 by two German scientists: Prof. Dr Günther Weitzel of Tübingen and Prof. Dr Eckhard Buddecke of Münster), both of whom I was later to collaborate with.

Reading their article, I was struck by how similar the pattern of development was between hens and humans: like us, hens exhibit marked arteriosclerosis in their old age (which in the case of hens is their third or fourth year); prior to that there is a gradual integration of fats into the inner walls of some of the arteries; in hens, plaques start building up in the abdominal section of the aorta, gradually spreading from there to other sections of the aorta and then to smaller blood vessels, as often happens in humans.

Furthermore, the likeness fitted my first two criteria exactly: the deposits of cholesterol and other fats in the arterial walls are similar both in fine tissue type and chemical composition to those in humans.

There would, therefore, be good reasons for choosing chickens and to feel that the results would help us in our understanding of the processes of arteriosclerotic development in humans. In addition to displaying the characteristics just described, hens were also inexpensive and easily available and, compared to us, very short-lived, which meant I could study the process speeded up, as it were.

There was also the third criterion to which to give our consideration – that of diet.

In the wild

It may come as a surprise to the reader that grain is not the original staple of hens. Charles Darwin identified the red jungle fowl, native to the forests of South-East Asia, as the originator of the modern stock from which our present-day domesticated chickens descended. In the jungle, where no grass seed would be found, these ancestral jungle fowl provided for themselves from the rich fauna of the forest.

In Roman times, chickens were used not so much to provide meat and eggs as to clean up the harvest fields from bugs and pests. Any chicken farmer will tell you how today's chickens, left to themselves, still like to scratch for their food, eating a variety of grubs, insects and worms, as well as seeds in season. Over time, it became customary to feed cereal grains to chickens on a regular basis and, currently, farmed chickens receive a diet consisting mainly and sometimes entirely of grain.

Thus, from having been more or less carnivorous in the wild, our domesticated fowl received increasing amounts of carbohydrate in their diet and nowadays live to a large extent on grain – not too unlike the story of our own humankind, perhaps? This parallel set me wondering whether this similarity in evolution meant that hens suffer similar disadvantages to health to those experienced by humans with the advent of cereal cultivation.

Was it too much to suppose that, in sharing the fruits of agriculture, hens and humans also shared the tendency to develop arteriosclerosis for the same reason? It was a thought! At any rate, this resemblance in original diet and subsequent dietetic history meant that chickens fulfilled my third criterion sufficiently to make them suitable subjects for my investigations. It was therefore chickens that I chose for the experiments detailed below.

Do not think, however, that in experimenting with hens I was planning to see confined, wretched and maltreated specimens, birds that were mere shadows of their former selves. On the contrary, my basic idea was to restore to the hens something akin to their original diet – which should of course make them healthier! Remember that our domestic hens were already prone to arteriosclerosis; the control diet, high in carbohydrate, would be no other than the usual hen feed to which they were already accustomed.

Setting up my chicken trials

My immediate object was to examine the role of carbohydrate in the genesis of arteriosclerosis. The underlying idea, by now familiar to the reader, was the potential damage done by food inappropriate to the particular species in question. In particular, I wanted to compare what happens to the blood vessels of hens when fed diets with different percentages of carbohydrate and fat – a pre-cereal, mainly animal food diet and a post-cereal, mainly plant food diet – and to monitor the resultant health of their arteries with regard to arteriosclerotic changes.

I had limited means at my disposal, having to provide most of the funds from my own pocket. However, as a physician hitherto completely unknown to him, I approached Prof. Weitzel. I found a ready listener when I suggested the explanation for the similar forms of arteriosclerosis seen in humans and hens might lie in the fact that, with the coming of cereals, both humans and chickens were led away from their original mode of nutrition. Interested in this notion, Prof. Weitzel generously placed at my disposal both his own experience and the facilities of his institute.

Prof. Buddecke lent me his assistance in the continuation and completion of the experiments, as did other colleagues. Later, Lävosan-Gesellschaft of Linz/Donau and the Ludwig-Boltzmann-Gesellschaft of Vienna and other local firms kindly offered me some funding, as did the Landesregierung of the province of Salzburg. I was profoundly grateful, as it enabled me to carry through the series of trials over the many years that they took to implement.

In setting up my experiments, I was lucky to find a good chicken breeder. At the time, I was living in Innkreis in Upper Austria and I had advertised in a local paper. I received a reply from someone who was living in the same district. This was Mr Fellner, a real chicken enthusiast who had held a high office in the government and who, now retired, was devoting his time to the keeping of poultry. We felt an immediate rapport and it was not long before we got down to business: Mr Fellner agreeing to oversee the day-to-day management of the chickens. So began the feeding experiment now to be described.

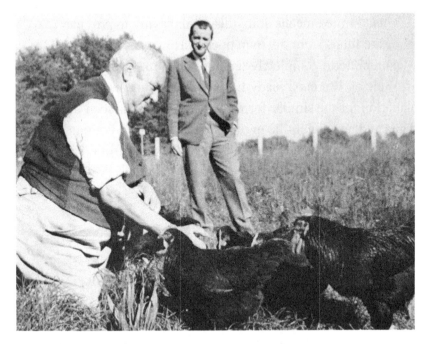

Dr Lutz visiting Mr. Fellner on his chicken farm.

I picked Rhode Island Reds for the trials, choosing as pure a strain as I could to minimise genetic variation and selecting birds that were equal in age and sex. The hens were treated the same in all ways but diet with conditions of rearing kept constant. I deliberately chose to avoid shutting the birds in small cages, allowing them plenty of space to run about. I also chose not to match their calorie intake, as I wanted the hens to be free to eat as much as they liked.

What I had in mind, as I said, was not to induce illness in any of the birds but rather to watch whether illness came about solely in consequence of the particular food they were eating. Nor did I want to speed up the process artificially. Therefore, we looked after the birds as best we could, being careful to ensure that their feed contained enough vitamins and minerals, and that it was sufficiently balanced to prevent any obvious nutritional deficiency. We then kept them for a good three years to give time for any arterial change to come about: if, that is, it came at all, without any inducement other than diet.

Feeding my chickens

The chicks came to me at six weeks old. I had hoped to take them from the start, but I was advised that the birds needed rearing for the first six weeks in the usual fashion. I then took over the control of the diet that the chicks were to be given. Professor Dr W. Wirths, of the Max Planck Institute in Dortmund, had done the calculations to ensure the correct composition of the feed in respect of protein, fat and carbohydrate and had also estimated the calorie content.

The chickens were divided into groups, which were given different levels of carbohydrate and fat in their feed, the birds with the highest ration of carbohydrate receiving the lowest amount of fat and vice versa; the protein content of the diet was kept fairly constant. The hens received the same mixture over the whole of the three years and they were, as I said, free to eat as much as they liked. Table 1 shows how the diet of the hens was put together.

The preliminary trial lasted from 1961-4. The chicks were divided into two groups: a high carbohydrate control group and a low carbohydrate group. In the subsequent larger trial from 1964-7, I added groups with a medium level of carbohydrate and the chicks were divided into six groups, each group with five chicks. Group I was my low carbohydrate group, Groups II and III the middle groups and Group VI the high carbohydrate Group. I had six groups so that we could compare a greater number of variables, but not every group was used in each experiment so Groups IV and V, which were cross-over groups, need not concern us as yet.

The 'high carbohydrate' group was my control group, the idea being to contrast the results of chickens fed a lower level of carbohydrate to those of this 'high' control group. Note the Group VI chickens were those being given feed with a carbohydrate level that by farming standards was normal for that time. On the other hand, Group I received a carbohydrate level similar to that of my own diet – I suppose this is why I often refer to these Group I birds 'my' chickens!

High and low are terms which are often used both in the sense of overall amount and also relative to the other ingredients of the diet. Thus 'high' means that roughly 75% of the hens' diet consisted of carbohydrate and the remaining 25% of protein and fat; conversely 'low' means 25% of the diet came from carbohydrate and the rest from protein and fat, whilst 'medium' worked out at 50/50. This is by dry weight (of grams of protein, fat and carbohydrate) as given in figure 20.2. From now on, I shall refer to these as the (high carbohydrate), (middle carbohydrate) and (low carbohydrate) birds respectively.

As you can see from Table 1, as regards carbohydrate, the terms 'high' and 'low' hold true as a description both as regards amount and percentage; we shall return to this tricky question in the next chapter.

I had decided to set up two middle groups: Group II with grain, Group III without grain but with fruit sugar (fructose) instead since, although I had a fair idea that too much carbohydrate was bad for the health, I was not sure whether it had the same deleterious effect from all sources. Looking back,

I feel that, for the sake of comparison, I should perhaps have had two high carbohydrate groups as well, but I did what I could with the means available at the time. My Group I birds had neither grain nor fruit sugar.

Group	Foodstuff	Quantity (g)	Protein (g)	Fat (g)	Carbo-hydrate (g)	kcal
I	Dried yeast	15	7.2	0.2	5.4	51.6
	Shrimps	7	1.1	0.1	0.2	6.1
	Cottage cheese	35	6.0	0.4	0.7	30.8
	Meat	50	8.0	11.5	-	140.5
	Skimmed milk	125	5.0	-	6.3	43.8
	TOTAL		27.3	12.2	12.6	272.8
II	Dried yeast	10	4.7	0.14	3.6	34.3
	Shrimps	4	0.6	0.06	0.12	3.5
	Cottage cheese	25	4.3	0.3	0.5	22.0
	Meat	35	5.6	8.1	-	101.0
	Wheat grains	35	4.1	0.7	24.3	127.1
	Skimmed milk	84	3.4	-	4.25	30.0
	TOTAL		22.7	9.30	32.77	317.9
III	Dried yeast	12	5.7	0.16	4.3	41.0
	Shrimps	5.6	0.88	0.08	0.16	4.9
	Cottage cheese	28	4.8	0.32	0.56	25.0
	Meat	40	6.4	8.3	-	112.0
	Skimmed milk	100	4.0	-	5.05	35.0
	Fructose	20	-	-	20.0	76.8
	TOTAL		21.8	10.9	30.1	294.7
VI	Dried yeast	10	4.9	0.13	3.6	34.4
	Shrimps	7	1.1	0.1	0.2	6.1
	Skimmed milk	125	5.0	-	6.3	43.8
	Wheat grains	120	14.0	2.4	83.2	435.3
	TOTAL		25.0	2.6	93.3	519.6

Table 1: The ingredients of the feed by weight of ingredient

All the hens were fed a basic mixture of dried yeast, shrimps, white cheese and skimmed milk. You will notice that, except the yeast, all these are animal foods. In fact, apart from the protein present in yeast (and in grain for those that received it), the protein we used for all groups was mainly animal protein and the fat mostly saturated fat. We were deliberately careful to limit both plant proteins and the quantity of unsaturated fat (iodine no. 59.2!) so that the outcome of the trials could not be wrongly ascribed to their influence.

My (low carbohydrate) chickens, as you see, were grain-free, getting what little carbohydrate they ate from the skimmed milk and the yeast; in addition to the basic foods, Group I and (middle carbohydrate) Groups II and IIII had meat (beef bone meal and pork) . The controls received wheat grain as their extra carbohydrate as did Group II.

Thus Group I received no grain at all and Group VI received no meat as such; the middle groups had more mixed diets. This was the nearest I could get to a Palaeolithic, Mesolithic and Neolithic equivalent!

My experiment was all set up and running. It was arranged that the results were to be independently analysed by staff from the biochemistry department at the University of Tübingen. I was swimming against the tide with my views on human nutrition and was now hoping to show that at least hens were on my side! But would my hens really come up to the mark? Would they show healthier arteries with less fatty deposits, less arteriosclerosis? I sincerely hoped so.

Happily, my results were beyond all expectation.

3 HEALTHIER ARTERIES

High or low?

Before we look at the results of my trials, let us pause to reflect on the confusion that both words and figures can lead us into. One needs to be so cautious of statistics: namely, figures of quantities and percentages frequently cause complications in the way we interpret data on human diets. It is so easy to bandy words about, especially phrases like 'high fat' or 'high protein'. In fact, I was tempted just now to ask whether my 'high fat, high protein' chickens would come up to the mark. But was the food of my Group 1 birds actually high in fat and protein or are these misleading terms?

The feed was deliberately mixed so that the chickens could not pick and choose and, say, just eat the shrimps. The proportions of the various foodstuffs therefore remained the same in the individual mixtures. The hens were allowed to eat as much as they liked and the feed taken was measured over the whole 38 months of the trial. The quantities given in grams in Table 1 in the last chapter represent the average amount the hens in each group ate on a daily basis during the trial period.

To illustrate my point about confusion, in Table 2, I give these figures again as percentages of the various ingredients. Take protein: the mixtures were made up with a fairly constant content of protein and it turned out that the hens of all groups ate more or less 25 g of protein a day. But, whereas the actual amount of protein the chickens received was fairly similar, as a percentage of their diet relative to fat and carbohydrate, the protein content, as you can see, varied considerably between

41

the groups. It is therefore questionable whether the diet had a stable or variable protein content!

Whether this 25 g of protein is considered a large amount or a little amount of protein depends, of course, on your viewpoint. The point is how do we describe the dietary balance of these two groups of hens? If we judge by actual amounts eaten, then we might conclude that both groups had, say, high protein feed. Yet, if we go by percentages of this very same ingredient, we might now draw the conclusion that Group I was high in protein (53%) but that Group VI was low in protein (21%) – another picture altogether and particularly ironic since we set up the trials to contrast the effects, not of eating different levels of protein, but of carbohydrate and fat!

Composition of Feed							
Group	Protein		Fats		Carbohydrate		Total calories
	g	%	g	%	g	%	
I	27.3	53	12.2	23	12.6	24	272
II	22.7	35	9.3	14.5	32.7	50.5	317
III	21.8	35	10.9	17	30.1	48	294
VI	25.0	21	2.6	2	93.3	77	446

Table 2: The composition of the feed given by weight and percentage of protein, carbohydrate and fat, and number of calories.

Likewise, from these figures we could truthfully say that Group I ate over four times as much fat as Group VI and about seven times less carbohydrate. Yet if we look at the same picture as percentages and do our sums again, it might be thought that the hens in Group I ate, not four times as much fat, but over eleven times as much as Group VI! The percentages would also seem to suggest that Group VI ate, not seven times as much carbohydrate, but merely three times that of Group I! Where indeed is the truth?

Differences in viewpoint can obviously lead to erroneous – and sometimes strange conclusions. Perhaps I should complicate the picture by breaking down these figures into percentages derived from calories? This is the habit of dieticians and it gives us different figures yet again. But what can we gather from knowing that Group I derives 18.7% of its total calories from carbohydrate, the middle group: 42.3% and control Group VI: 73%? Can we know what such percentages look like – either in the chicken coop or on the dinner plate?

This problem of low and high is a trap few of us have not fallen into at some time and I am no exception. My own diet is very modest in the actual amount of carbohydrate which I consume: that is it is low in carbohydrate compared to average intake and low relative to the percentages of fat and protein eaten. However, describing it as a low carbohydrate diet leaves it open to imputations of being higher than normal in protein content – though this is not necessarily the case any more than it is with my hens and it is likewise with the fat content.

Take heed those of you who indiscriminately label low carbohydrate diets as high fat, high protein diets and first ascertain what your modest neighbour actually eats!

Perhaps you can now see why I chose to specify a particular number of bread units (grams of carbohydrate) a day for my patients, advised weighing scales and gave them tables and diet sheets, so that they could manage work out the diet themselves in their own kitchens. And, also why I allowed free choice as to quantity of protein and fat?

Now let us look and see what happened to the different groups of hens and whether the composition of their feed did in fact make any difference to their health.

The results of my chicken experiments

During both series of my chicken trials, I made some general observations as to the overall health of the hens. For it soon became apparent that the chickens in Group I fared differently to those in the control Group VI. During the first trial, even to the casual observer, the difference in the feathers of the hens was noticeable. The Group I (low carbohydrate) hens had glossy, sleek plumage in contrast to which Group VI hens had dull-looking feathers, which lacked the shine of healthy birds.

Even whilst they were still chicks, there were differences: for example, Group I birds grew more slowly, and they did not appear to put on fat in the way Group VI birds did. As they grew older, the Group I birds stayed slim and fit – if you can call chickens slim! By this I mean that they showed a slow and steady weight gain, which seemed to be more muscle than fat. It was not that one group put on weight, while the other did not: the weight of the two groups did not differ much. It was more that Group VI birds had more fat and less muscle and were less fit generally, whilst Group I birds were sturdier.

Since I did these trials, I have heard a lot about the sufferings of present-day chickens and their bone problems – their bandy legs and sometimes their inability to even stand. We did not measure bone density in our birds but, from the way they ran about happily, I certainly had no worries for my (low carbohydrate) hens in this respect. I was interested to see whether this externally apparent general fitness was accompanied by better arterial health.

Although our examination for arteriosclerosis was to be only after the third year, in the first series Prof. Weitzel did an earlier examination of the fats present in the arteries of some of the hens. The results of this initial analysis were encouraging. You will recall that arteriosclerosis starts, for whatever reason, with weakness or damage to the endothelium and that the first obvious stage of the process is an integration of lipids into the arterial walls. (Please note that I am using the words 'fats' and 'lipids' fairly interchangeably, as is general in common parlance.)

Well, in hens too, similar weakness or damage is followed by the proliferation of smooth muscle cells, which fill with lipids and appear as raised fatty striae (streaks) on the inside wall of the artery. Later, come thick fibrous plaques filled with cell debris and encapsulated by so-called foam cells (the lipid-filled smooth muscle cells), which contain cholesterol and may eventually become calcified. In our trials, we concentrated on the amount of fat in the artery walls and the formation of plaques as indices of arteriosclerosis.

What Prof. Weitzel found after two years was that the arteriosclerotic process had already begun, and that fat was already being put down in the arteries of some of the hens. The inequality of its distribution between the two groups was striking for a lot less fat had found its way into the artery walls of the (low carbohydrate) hens than into those of the (high carbohydrate) control group. This was in spite Group I birds eating more animal fat. From this initial investigation, I knew that I was on the right lines.

The adult human aorta is about one and a half feet long and an inch wide and, with arteriosclerosis, fatty striae and plaques can easily be seen with the naked eye. The aortas of hens are, of course, a lot narrower but such degenerative changes are still visible to macroscopic inspection. This visual examination with the naked eye was one of the ways we tested for arteriosclerosis.

When the hens were examined in this way after the full three years, in some of the control group we found pronounced atheroma with its deep yellow colouring and lipid streaks. In the photograph below, in the aorta fragment (upper) taken from one of the Group VI hens, a porridge-like, fatty plaque, characteristic of advanced arteriosclerosis, is distinctly visible , whereas there is no such plaque in the aorta taken from a group I hen, which is smoother. The lower fragment of aorta of the Group I hen was much lighter yellow colour.

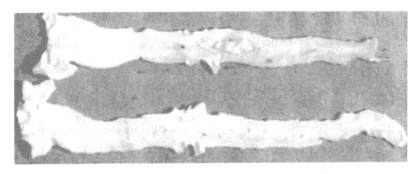

Aortas of hens after three years: above, on the control diet with very little fat; below, Group I on the low carbohydrate diet with a moderate amount of mainly saturated fat.

From these typical specimens, it can be seen that the arterial health of the (lower carbohydrate, higher fat) hens compares very favourably to that of the (higher carbohydrate, lower fat) birds. This confirmed the same trend that was seen earlier: namely that the arteries of the (low carbohydrate) birds were distinctly healthier than those of the (high carbohydrate) birds. Frau G. Andresen of Tübingen did the visual analyses and was very experienced in such work. I remember her once telling me:

> "Dr Lutz, I have examined the aortas of many thousands of chickens and, in all the years I have being doing my job, I have never seen these blood vessels with less arteriosclerosis. In fact, I have never seen chickens with such healthy arteries as those of your own hens!"

So, to me, there was no doubt as to the results!

However, after what I said above about high and low percentages and amounts, I now have the daunting task of presenting the numerical details of my own results! These were independently analysed by staff at Tübingen University and found to be statistically viable. Any details of the results not given here can be found in an article in the *Zeitschrift für Ernährungswissenschaft* (journal of nutritional science) in 1969 that I subsequently wrote with Prof. Buddecke and Frau Andresen. Translated, the article is entitled 'Investigations into the Influence of a long-term low carbohydrate diet on the Arteriosclerosis of hens.'

In order to compare the results of the visual examination, the severity of the arteriosclerosis was expressed on a scale of 0 to 6, with 0 showing no obvious degenerative change and 6, severe arteriosclerosis. In the first series of experiments, Group I hens rated: 1.5, 0.0, 0.5, 0.0, 0.5, and Group VI: 6.0, 2.0, 6.0, 6.0, 0.0, 1.0, 4.5. In the second series, done from 1964-7, Group I rated: 1.0, 0.5, 3.5, 0.5, 0.0, and Group VI: 1.0, 1.5,

3.0, 4.5, 4.5. If we add these figures together, they average: 0.8 for Group I, and 3.3 for Group VI, demonstrating that the arteriosclerosis was far less severe in my (low carbohydrate) hens than in the controls.

In terms of identifying the level of arteriosclerosis, the results derived by looking with the naked eye or under magnification reflect fairly accurately the results obtained by chemical analysis of the fats present in the arterial walls, although there are some anomalies. By various chemical procedures, the fat content of the arteries is measured with the arteries in a fresh state and then in a dried state; it is done both ways as the results come out slightly differently, though the differences are not such that they affected the significance of the overall results. These tests were carried out after the second and larger trial was completed in 1967.

What did the biochemical analyses show? They confirmed the pronouncement of the visual inspection – that there was clearly more deposition of fats in the artery walls of the control group than of the other groups and clearly more arteriosclerosis present.

If we start by taking Groups I and VI, the final chemical analysis showed an unmistakable difference in the amount of fats present in the artery walls: that the amount of total lipids present, as well as total cholesterol and phospholipids was lower in the Group I (low carbohydrate) birds than in the Group VI (high carbohydrate) birds. This can be seen in the bar diagram in Table 3 below.

Thus the birds that were eating a relatively low level of carbohydrate had a relatively low level of fat in their artery walls and, conversely, the birds that were eating a relatively high level of carbohydrate had a relatively high level of deposited or integrated fats in their arteries. On the face of it, there certainly seemed to be a correlation between quantity of dietary carbohydrate eaten and the amount of fat present in the arteries of our hens.

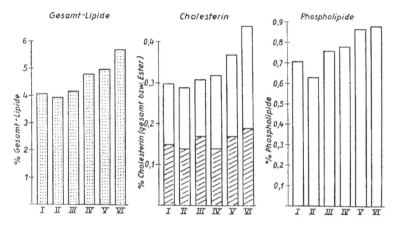

Table 3: Total lipids, cholesterol and phospholipids in the aortas of the experimental birds given by percentage of fresh weight.

However, the hens were also eating protein and fat, not just carbohydrates. The protein level being similar, we must next look at the incidence of arteriosclerosis in relation to the intake of dietary fat. According to the tenets of the fat theory one would expect the presence of more fat in diet of the hens to augment arteriosclerotic change, so it was particularly striking that the results showed no such relationship. On the contrary, the Group I hens that ate more fat – and remember it was mostly saturated fat – had on average less arteriosclerosis at the end of the three years and, conversely, the Group IV that ate less fat had more arteriosclerosis.

Judging from the results of Groups I and VI alone one might conclude: the less dietary fat, the more arteriosclerosis, just as one might conclude: the more carbohydrate, the more arteriosclerosis. However, it was not quite that simple, at least in any absolute sense. Groups II and III, the middle groups did fairly well and certainly better than I expected. In fact, in terms of specific fats present in the arteries, there is no group that has the lowest absolute values on all counts, though all groups showed lower values than the control group that was receiving the so-called normal chicken feed.

From the bar diagram in Table 3, it would seem that Group II (which had feed with a medium level of fat and carbohydrate, including some wheat grain), did even better than Group I and this is so when we compare the fat content of the arteries by percentage of the fresh weight of the aortas.

The situation changes when we compare the same groups by percentage of dry weight, and again by visual rating, as can be seen in Table 4, which gives the measurements of fats found in the arterial walls of the hens in the main trial as percentages compared to the control group. In this table, Control Group VI with its customarily high carbohydrate feed is counted as 100% for easy comparison. That total lipids are lower in Groups I to V than those of Group VI can be seen from columns one and two.

From these tables, one can see that the composition of the feed influenced the amount of fat present in the aortas of the hens, but that there was variation in the proportion of the different fats deposited.

Gr.	Relative % (fresh weight)				Relative % (dry weight)				Relative % (total lipids)		
	Lipids	Cholesterol		Phos	Lipids	Cholesterol		Phos	Cholesterol		Phos
	Total	Total	Free		Total	Total	Free		Total	Free	
I	71.3	68.1	78.9	80.6	79.0	82.2	83.1	89.3	103.5	105.9	113.4
II	69.1	65.9	73.6	71.5	84.3	82.2	86.7	88.0	97.2	102.0	104.5
III	75.2	70.4	89.4	86.3	80.6	75.8	96.3	92.8	93.9	119.1	115.2
IV	84.4	72.7	73.6	88.6	89.5	78.4	79.5	94.1	87.6	88.3	105.0
V	87.4	84.0	89.4	98.8	90.1	87.6	89.1	101.8	96.9	99.4	113.1
VI	100	100	100	100	100	100	100	100	100	100	100

Table 4: Relative percentage of lipids: Groups I–V are compared to the Control Group VI (phos = phospholipids)

Probably the best way of getting a good idea of the overall results as the incidence of arteriosclerosis is to study Table 5. This gives the results of the visual examination of the hens of all six groups. From this, one can see that Group VI hens (high carbohydrate, low fat) showed significantly more damage to their arteries than the hens in Group I (mainly protein + fat, with no grain)

Group	Average	Incidence of Arteriosclerosis
I	1.1	1.0, 0.5, 3.5, 0.5, 0.0
II	1.6	1.5, 2.5, 0.5, 2.0
III	2.2	2.0, 3.5, 1.0
IV	0.9	0.5, 1.5, 0.5, 1.0
V	2.4	1.0, 3.0, 4.0, 1.5
VI	2.9	1.0, 1.5, 3.0, 4.5, 4.5

Table 5: The incidence of arteriosclerosis in all six groups as judged by the naked eye

If we compare Group II (middle carbohydrate with grain) and Group III (middle carbohydrate with D-fructose), the grain group fared marginally better. Taking Groups I, II, III and VI and leaving aside the cross-over Groups IV and V, which formed part of a different line of enquiry, these figures show how the rise in the severity of arteriosclerosis parallels the rise in the carbohydrate content of the food. It also shows how this is inversely related to the fat content.

Was it, then, the absence of enough dietary fat or the presence of too much carbohydrate that served to promote arteriosclerosis? With two variables, one can never be totally sure which one is causal or whether it is the mixture of the two! Yet I had reason to think the finger of suspicion pointed at carbohydrate.

Too late to change?

One question that interested me in those days was whether, after a childhood and beyond spent eating carbohydrate with abandon, it was still worth cutting down on carbohydrates. Was it too late by then to cut down the risk of heart attacks? As I myself had spent something like half my life eating unrestricted carbohydrates, I had a personal interest in the question of whether it was too late to cut down – a positive result from trials would certainly be reassuring!

This was where Groups IV and V came in. In second trial, Group IV was fed like the (high carbohydrate) Group VI for the first year and then like (low carbohydrate) Group I for the remaining two years. Group V was fed the other way round, i.e. like Group I for one year and then like Group VI for two. Details of the results are given in the Tables 3-5 and in

Table 5 you can see how well cross-over Group IV fared in comparison to Group V. This was just the reassurance I needed!

In summary our findings were as follows: if hens switched from a high to a low carbohydrate diet after the first third of their lives (Group IV), this still exercised a marked protective effect against developing arteriosclerosis later in their lives. Switching to a high intake after one year (Group V) was, on the other hand, aggravating, though even this initial period of low intake gave a small amount of protection. These observations were potentially important.

Individual variation

A further issue raised by my research was the question of individual variation. Results are never uniform and one always has to allow for a certain measure of intrinsic variation. As Matt Ridley says:

> 'Variation is an inherent and integral part of the human – or indeed any – genome.'

> Ridley (1999)

However, I was still struck by the considerable variation in the development of arteriosclerosis shown by the hens eating the same amount of carbohydrate – and this despite being chosen for their pure strain to eliminate genetic variation as far as possible.

The range of individual variation tends to be obscured by citing averages so I have given the results for each hen in both trials. The tables given earlier, show that the atheroma in the (high carbohydrate) hens ranged from none to very severe. It was obviously possible for some hens to eat the control diet and not suffer severe consequences: in fact, one of them did so with no signs of arterial damage at all. Arteriosclerosis in hens was not therefore an inevitable consequence of a low fat, high carbohydrate diet. I have long wondered why some individuals – whether fowl or human – are less affected by, or even escape entirely from the general pattern.

If we look again at the figures for the all the Group VI hens, it can be seen that the group as a whole contained more individual hens with a middling to severe occurrence than with little. Likewise, amongst the hens fed little carbohydrate as a group, most of the (low carbohydrate) hens had a low rating, and none had more than a middling amount of arteriosclerosis. A general pattern had emerged: since, though not an inevitable consequence of a high carbohydrate diet, my work showed that arterial damage in the form of arteriosclerosis was more likely to happen than not.

Thus, despite individual variation, on a diet severely curtailing carbohydrate, there was not a single incidence amongst these hens of severe arteriosclerosis. This supports my conclusion that a diet containing a meagre ration of carbohydrate, together with a moderate amount of fat and protein, exerted a marked protective effect on the health of the chickens in respect of arteriosclerosis.

Judging by my trials, a diet based mainly on animal protein and fat with little carbohydrate offered the hens significant protection of their arteries and, by implication, from heart attacks and strokes. (Yes, hens do have heart attacks, sadly the more so in these days of intensive cereal feeding.) Thus, a diet more akin in composition to the hen's original diet in the wild did produce birds with healthier arteries.

These results were indeed gratifying. Naturally, the full extent to which these findings apply to us was not possible for me to say. However, as the prevailing dietary advice for human beings is to eat little fat but much carbohydrate, at this stage I could only conclude that such advice would render no service to the health of hens!

4 FINDINGS TO PONDER

The influence of diet on calorie intake

The relationship between carbohydrate and calorie intake has been the subject of on-going debate among scientific circles for many years. In this regard, we made an interesting observation during the trials. As I said, we mixed up the ingredients of their food in the agreed proportions ourselves and the chickens were free to eat as much as they chose to eat.

Fat having just over twice the number calories as carbohydrates, gram for gram the low carbohydrate feed was much higher in calories than the high carbohydrate feed. One might have thought that, since the feed of Group I with its higher fat content was richer, those hens would merely eat less overall and that the other groups would take proportionately more feed to cover their energy needs. In this way, calorie consumption would have been more or less the same between the groups. Yet this was not so.

The hens that consumed more carbohydrate had a higher intake of calories. Food intake was strictly measured throughout the experiments and it was calculated that the hens receiving 18.7% of their calories from carbohydrate ate 273 calories per bird per day, the middle groups, which on average received 42.3% of their calories from carbohydrate took 318, whereas the group receiving 73.7% of their calories from carbohydrate averaged 520 calories – and this, remember, was voluntary intake.

Even after allowing for the extra calories needed for the difference in egg-laying between the two groups, it still held true that the more carbohydrate in their food, the more the hens chose to eat and the more calories they consumed. In fact, the calorific value of the actual amount of feed consumed was in inverse proportion to the calorific value of the feed itself. (Per 100 g of dry weight, the calorific value of the feed was: 523.6 kcal for Group I, 490 kcal for Group II, 458 for Group III and 369 for Group VI.)

The content of the food seemed to influence the number of calories the hens chose to eat. It was as if control Group VI (high-carbohydrate, low-fat) hens were in effect overeating. In humans, overeating is often ascribed to poor self-esteem or anxiety but I think we can safely rule out emotional influences here: comfort eating or worry nibbling seemed scarcely applicable to hens and certainly not to our own groups of unstressed, free-running chickens.

So why were the (high carbohydrate) hens eating more food than the others? Was it a bit like fat youngsters eating biscuits – the more they ate the more they craved? Was the insulin mechanism of the control Group VI affected by their carbohydrate intake in the same way as that of my young people? I did not measure blood sugar response in my experimental birds.

Why does this matter? Well, in our trials, the incidence of arteriosclerosis paralleled both the carbohydrate and the calorie intake, so it could be thought that it was the number of calories per se that was responsible for this increase. But as the hens chose their own quantity of food, the inference was that it was the effect of eating so much carbohydrate that was self-perpetuating, with the calorie intake incidental. This suggests that it was the high level of carbohydrate intake that was primarily implicated in arteriosclerotic change, with increased appetite and increased calorie intake as secondary factors – a view, which was later corroborated by follow-up work done by colleagues, as we shall now see.

I encounter Professor Jürgen Schole

By the time I finished my chicken-feeding trials, it was already 1969, the year after I had moved to Salzburg to work. Medically speaking, things are a little different when you move from a rural practice to the city for here there was more specialism: for example, fat children were likely to be seen by the paediatrician and people with multiple sclerosis or epilepsy by the neurologist. Nevertheless, as a consultant in internal medicine, I still saw patients with a wide range of conditions.

By this time ten years had elapsed since I started using carbohydrate restriction as a therapeutic tool. I had made many observations in regard to carbohydrate and the endocrine system, especially as regards obese juveniles but I was still pondering how my diverse observations could be explained. The chicken trials had been successful in showing a link between carbohydrate intake and arteriosclerosis in hens and had brought further thought-provoking and unexpected extra findings along the way.

Nevertheless, my experiments were already attracting criticism. An acquaintance of mine, a vet, told me that a particular professor disapproved of my method of conducting my research. My critic turned out to be none other than biochemist Prof. Dr Jürgen K. Schole from the School of Veterinary Medicine at Hanover University, Germany.

I am pleased to report that, after an exchange of letters, Prof. Schole suggested we meet in Munich. This we did and the meeting marked the beginning of a life-long personal friendship. Moreover, it was to be the beginning of a lasting and fruitful interchange of ideas between us. Many years later, in the 1980's, we were to collaborate on a book: *Regulationskrankheiten* (diseases of hormonal regulation).

Let us remain for a moment in 1969, the year when I met Prof. Schole in Munich. For it was soon obvious that, albeit from a different angle, we shared a fascination for hormonal behaviour. At the time of our first encounter, Prof. Schole and his colleagues had been doing detailed research work on the effect of carbohydrates on the metabolism of warm-bloodied animals and this was of particular interest to me.

Schole had focussed on the endocrinal mechanisms that regulated efficient energy exchange and saw knowledge of the way hormones work at molecular level as not only fundamental to health but the basis for understanding the diseases to do with hormonal regulation and with the body's adaptation to stress. As I listened to him talk about his research and expound his ideas, certain things he said struck a real chord in me.

Nature is apt to use a successful biological mechanism over and over again and, as I said previously, we humans share a lot of our physiological processes with our fellow creatures. Just as there were inferences from my chicken experiments that were worth exploring in relation to human health so, too, I felt that the results of Schole's veterinary research would most likely have significance for us and our human health problems.

I myself, as you know, had noted that a high intake of carbohydrate seemed as foreign to the metabolism of hens as to that of humans and also seemed to lead to similar disturbances in health. Now, here was a professor of biochemistry who was suggesting that the hormonal balance of any warm-bloodied animal was likely to be upset by excessive carbohydrate intake.

This, of course, immediately caught my imagination. Moreover, the endocrine hormones, in which I myself had discerned a certain pattern in obese youth, turned out to be the very hormones that were central to the observations made by Schole. He, too, found raised insulin levels and disturbed sex hormone levels, together with a depressed level of growth hormone and elevated levels of adrenal and thyroid hormones, all seemingly implicated in the development of arteriosclerosis.

Schole was later to give me credit for my own observations on humans in the foreword to the ninth German edition of my book *Leben ohne Brot* (Life without Bread), which was translated into English in 1986 as *Dismantling a Myth: the role of fat and carbohydrates in our diet.*

Lutz has identified very nicely the 'regulatory diseases', which respond to carbohydrate restriction. Furthermore, he was the first to describe the endocrine events that underlie these disorders. Generally, his view coincides with the basic metabolic regulation we have postulated based on experimental results.

I would like, in my turn, to pay tribute to my late friend, Jürgen Schole, as the one who gave cogency to these observations of mine by providing me with insight into the mechanism of hormonal equilibrium.

But back to my chicken trials and the criticism they had attracted. Apparently, giving the chickens a free run did not provide rigorous enough scientific control. I personally disapproved of caging birds and thought it was a better idea to keep hens in a good condition. In fact, I was rather pleased that my experimental birds – those on a low carbohydrate diet, of course – had exhibited such splendid physique. My approach to calories also did not meet approval.

Anyway, one of the results of our initial meeting was that Prof. Schole, himself, felt he wanted to show – he said more scientifically – whether the corrupting effect that carbohydrate had on the metabolism might contribute to the development of arteriosclerosis. He was therefore keen to do his own chicken experiments. This he did together with Professors P. Sallmann and G. Harisch, who were also from the School of Veterinary Medicine at Hanover University.

These experiments were unlike my own in method, composition of feed, the caging of the birds and even the various factors measured. However, their focus was, as I said, arteriosclerosis and they had five groups of hens over two years which received different amounts of carbohydrate. As to the benefit of carbohydrate restriction in reducing the incidence of arteriosclerosis, it was gratifying that their results did indeed confirm the results of my own trial.

Was it the carbohydrate or the calories, though? Well, all Schole's hens were deliberately given the same number of calories so that there was no confusion here. With calories held constant, the results showed clearly that the lower the amount of carbohydrate eaten, the less arteriosclerosis developed; conversely the more carbohydrate the hens ate, the higher the amount of arteriosclerosis in their arteries.

The spontaneous arteriosclerosis of chickens is definitely less developed when carbohydrates are replaced by isocaloric amounts of fat or protein. The quality of the fats is less important.

(Sallmann, Harisch and Schole, 1976)

As to obesity, it was also interesting that the study found that, given the same number of calories and roughly the same amount of protein, it was those hens that derived more of their calories from carbohydrate, rather than from the fat in their feed, which grew fat. As Schole said himself, his results gave the lie to the old saying that 'calories are just calories'.

A relationship between insulin and atheroma in humans had already been suggested not only by me but also, amongst others, by Stout and Vallance-Owen in 1969 and John Yudkin in 1971. From the perspective of endocrinology, Schole now added his study-based observation that the more carbohydrate the hens consumed, the higher their insulin levels and the demonstrably lower their level of growth hormone.

This hormonal situation, he argued as I had done, weakened their resistance to stress (including rendering them more liable to infection) and to tissue damage resulting in arteriosclorotic changes. Fat was not implicated in that it does not significantly raise the level of insulin in the blood: calories from fat, he said, only worsened arterial damage when eaten in conjunction with plentiful carbohydrates. Schole concluded that replacing carbohydrate by fat or protein lowers the insulin level, thus reducing the tendency to arteriosclerotic changes.

The protective effect of eating more natural food

Let us now explore further this concept of protection. In my own chicken trials, my (low carbohydrate) hens, which were allowed to eat as much of the feed as they liked, freely chose to eat fewer calories. This, in itself, seemed to offer them a certain protection from overeating. Was this the satiating factor of enough fat or the absence of an insulin-led false hunger?

Carbohydrate restriction, as Schole noted, had also benefited the health of my own hens by protecting them from obesity. That a meagre carbohydrate ration protects hens from obesity was shown by its absence in our Group I (low carbohydrate) chickens in contrast to those eating the highest ration of carbohydrate. We found that as the Group VI hens went on eating carbohydrates, they quite simply grew fatter.

Now, I say they 'quite simply' grew fatter but observing that Group VI grew fatter was not the end of the story: for whilst the Group VI mainly grain-fed hens grew fatter, they did not grow heavier than the birds fed mainly animal food. It was more that the Group VI hens put on fat at the expense of muscle and other body-building materials. In fact, they displayed poor physique generally: their musculature was poor and fatty, their tissue quality generally below par and their feathers dull.

Moreover, this was not the only disturbance they exhibited in their health. They also showed signs of further problems with their hormonal equilibrium. The reproduction of Group VI hens was affected: egg-laying was speeded up and the climacteric delayed; at the end of the third year of life, the ovaries of these hens still held many preformed eggs.

Not so for my Group I birds! The situation for them was characterised, not just by the absence of the negative, but by a plus in that these hens seemed to be faring very well in every respect. As far as we could tell, the hens fed mainly on protein and fat were altogether healthier: namely, these fowl, which received less than one fifth of their calories from carbohydrate, were sleeker, had fine glossy plumage and more muscle. Moreover, by the end of their lives, the ovaries of these hens had completely atrophied, which is as it should be.

Thus, the protective effect of carbohydrate restriction was far more extensive than that which I had envisaged when setting up my experiments. These birds, which ate no corn at all, displayed medal-winning physique. This is not just my pride speaking, for they did actually win medals – my keeper was himself so proud of their condition that he exhibited them at poultry shows!

I am reminded by mention of my keeper of a chance observation made during our trials. I had told Mr Fellner that, as one of the perks of the job, he could keep the eggs from my low carbohydrate hens. Seeing the lovely condition of these birds, I asked him in conversation one day how he had enjoyed the eggs. "What eggs?" he had asked with a wry smile. It was in this way that I discovered that there was a surprise in store in the field of reproduction.

A surprise in store

In the wild, birds generally lay a nestful of eggs once or twice annually. This is, of course, normal since they can only hope to rear a limited number of progeny. In the wild, a hen, too, would lay a nestful of eggs once or twice annually; on its natural food, which would be in effect a low carbohydrate diet, it would begin laying relatively late and it would cease to reproduce at an early age.

We humans have domesticated the wild hen over the course of several thousand years and have come to realise that feeding carbohydrate leads to the desired egg production. In my younger days in rural Austria, it was the practice on old farmsteads for the farmer's wife to look after the poultry. Asked why she feeds her hens with grain when there is plenty of animal food (beetles, worms, grubs, insects of all kinds) to be found in field and farmyard, she would at once reply that they will not lay sufficiently otherwise.

I had not foreseen that, once this impetus to increased egg production was removed, things would change either so rapidly or so dramatically. I now learnt that the laying pattern of my Group I birds had changed: our low carbohydrate, domesticated birds were laying less frequently than those fed on grain and were laying far fewer eggs: approximately 30 as compared to 200 eggs per year. Furthermore, the Group I fowl commenced laying at a later age and their eggs were smaller and paler in colour.

I received a further surprise when, after the eggs of our (low carbohydrate) fed hens were allowed to hatch, we gave the resulting chicks the normal, high carbohydrate feed. Knowing that grain-feeding encourages laying, one might have expected that the chicks, once full-grown, would exhibit the same characteristic laying pattern as other (high carbohydrate) hens, rather than that of their low carbohydrate mothers. But this was not found to be the case: namely, even the offspring of the (low carbohydrate) mothers began to lay later than comparable members of their species, the eggs – like those of their mothers – being smaller and much fewer in number.

So what was going on? It seemed that my Group I birds had immediately reverted to their 'primitive' state, a state akin to that of their sisters in the wild, thereby revealing a more natural hormonal pattern of reproduction. The timely atrophy of their ovaries of these hens was further evidence of this. Moreover, our experiments showed that when the birds were deprived of their habitual amount of carbohydrate, they not only immediately reverted to reproductive behaviour characteristic of wild birds, but they then clung to it with such tenacity that it took several generations on a high carbohydrate diet before their hormonal apparatus returned to the state which we regard as normal!

A more natural pattern of reproduction

We expect chickens to lay well and even breed them selectively to do so: the offspring of the 'good layers' therefore tend also to be 'good layers', the assumption being that we have a modern sort of chicken to whom such prolific egg-laying is natural. Underlying this is the further assumption that, somewhere along the line, there has been a changeover to a new metabolic programme. The domestic hen has gone through an estimated 2-3,000 generations on increasing amounts of carbohydrate, so one might well think this time enough for a hen's genetic material to adapt to its new type of diet.

Yet, judging by the results of my trials, no such process has taken place. The speed at which my low carbohydrate birds had 'reverted to type', i.e. to the behaviour of wild birds, tended to suggest a certain long-term stability of the genome in relation to both reproductive behaviour and to their original food: that the metabolism of the domesticated hen was, to all intents and purposes, still the same as it had been before domestication. In other words, the behaviour of the wild bird was not only still inherent in their genetic make-up, but accessible within one generation.

One to two nests a year would therefore represent physiological normality. In this scenario, constant egg-laying has to be seen as a newly-learnt characteristic, which would, of course, be reflected in the genes – not as the healthful result of changing behaviour through a change of species, but rather as an 'acquired characteristic', as postulated by the French naturalist, Lamarck. If one to two nests a year was normal, constant egg-laying can be viewed as the result of the corrupting effect of carbohydrate on the hen's metabolism. In this light, too, we can see the passing on of this enhanced egg-laying capacity by the (high carbohydrate) hens to their daughters as acquired characteristics being passed on to the next generation, a process that was heightened by selection for egg-laying capacity. In this case, might not the acquired characteristics passed on to the hens' offspring include the disturbance of reproductive hormones?

As it was not the focus of my trials, I did not measure the hormone levels in my hens. But given the hormonal impetus needed to lay eggs, surely the (high carbohydrate) controls, which laid copious eggs, had considerably elevated levels of gonadotrophins (therefore of oestrogens and progesterone)? Surely, too, once no longer coerced by the abnormal stimulus of extra carbohydrate in their diet, the return of the (low carbohydrate) hens to an egg-laying pattern of wild birds showed that their sex hormone levels had returned to normal?

To sum up this point: the (high carbohydrate) birds exhibited an unnatural pattern of egg-laying (a sign of hormonal corruption), which they then passed on to their chicks. The (low carbohydrate) birds, on the other hand, not only became healthy within their own lifetime but bore healthy chicks with no such legacy. Put together with the increased tendency to arteriosclerosis and obesity amongst the former group, the implications of these observations are, I feel, profound.

If a similar scenario were to exist for human beings, by limiting dietary carbohydrate might it not be possible for parents at least to some extent to protect the next generation against some of the so-called diseases of civilisation, diseases to which even fowl were prone on a high enough carbohydrate diet? It is a question worth asking!

Looking back at my chickens

My experiments were not perfect, I know. Years later, when I look back at my experiments, I think I perhaps gave too little attention to the middle groups. For instance, the cross-over experiments were promising, but I only tried them by switching between the diet of Groups I and VI. I do not know if swapping after one year to a moderate intake of carbohydrate would have had the beneficial effect that swapping to a low intake of carbohydrate had and likewise with fat intake. I doubt it, but you never know without trying it.

Also, since the information on egg production came from a chance observation of my keeper, I do not have similar information on Groups II and III. Nor did we do any follow-up studies of the chicks of the low carbohydrate mothers in respect of arteriosclerosis. It would be a fascinating project to see whether one could overcome arteriosclerosis by breeding it out, as it were. If the chicks of the low carbohydrate mothers were fed a low carbohydrate diet for several generations, true they would not offer commercially viable egg production, but would their arteries then be as clean as whistles? It is possible. And would it have made a difference if, during the first six weeks, the chicks had not been given the standard feed, but had started life as we meant them to continue? Or if we had omitted skimmed milk and concentrated more on grubs and beetles – i.e. if the feed had been even more similar to their ancient diet and lower still in carbohydrate? There is plenty of scope for further research, though I understand that, in some countries, there are now legal restrictions as to feeding any animal food to these once carnivorous birds. This would only be allowable therefore if the grubs and beetles were live!

Over the years, I have had with me neither a team of research assistants nor enough interest from the universities to explore all the variables myself. I must therefore leave this further research to others.

A fundamental misunderstanding

The positive results of my chicken experiments had given me the confidence I needed to pursue what was then – and to some extent still is – a highly contentious dietary regime with my patients. For over forty years I have treated many thousands of patients for a wide variety of complaints, complaints often referred to as the diseases of civilisation.

As a doctor, my prescription of course varied to suit individual patients but, in the main, I used a diet containing carbohydrate in the region of 60 – 72 g daily and with as much protein and fat as the patient chose to eat. My results were often good and detailed descriptions of my work can be found in my books and articles.

All this supported my long-held basic thesis that we have not changed sufficiently since our Ice-Age origins to fully cope with the coming of agriculture, let alone with, shall we say today's dietary recommendations? Our forebears, like those of modern chickens, were predominantly eaters of animal food:

that is to say, animal protein and animal fat would have been the main components of their diet, namely the very substances to which our metabolism was – and, I think, still is – adapted. All living things, plants and animals, contain protein, carbohydrate and fat, though in very different proportions. Of necessity, in some parts of the world, people have had to derive some, or even most of these nutrients from plant food, supplemented by whatever animal protein and fat was or is available. In these areas we may see a different pattern of disease, conditions characterised by a 'too little' rather than a 'too much'.

However, a cuisine based on shortage of food per se, is a far cry from the growing abundance of easily available food that has taken place elsewhere. During both World Wars, the incidence of our civilised diseases lessened, but remember that there was less carbohydrate, less fat as well as less protein. Since then, there has been a massive surge in carbohydrate consumption relative to fat and protein and especially of refined, ready-made commercially produced foods.

The rise of the so-called food industry, with its often cheap, sugar and starch-laden products, has made it much easier to over-consume carbohydrates and over-consumption of carbohydrates is, I feel sure, at the root of many of our chronic degenerative diseases of today. The problem created by the shift from our original diet has been compounded by the fat theory, which is now embedded in our nutritional guidelines with the advice to curtail even natural fats, together with its accompanying scaremongering.

In consequence, our diseases of civilisation have soared to almost epidemic proportions. Thus, ironically, the fat theory has accomplished the very opposite of its original intent:

namely that the incidence of diseases such as obesity, diabetes, heart infarcts, osteoarthritis, gout, strokes and cancer has not honoured the widespread renunciation of fat that has taken place throughout the western world.

A stumbling block

A real stumbling block to progress is the seeming revision of our basic biology. Over the last sixty years or so, there has gradually come about a fundamental misinterpretation of our physiological needs. This is to believe that because nowadays our primary internal fuel tends, of necessity, to be sugar, it follows that sugar is the metabolically correct primary fuel and that this corresponds to the nature's inherent design for us. It does not.

This new pattern is therefore beginning to be seen and accepted as the biological norm, not as the desperate measure it is, which the body has had to adopt to protect itself from constant overdose. In health, the endocrine system is self-regulating in such a smooth and inconspicuous way that most of us would not even know we have one. Yet today, the words blood sugar and insulin are on everyone's lips. Diabetes is all too often seen as an unfortunate illness to be managed by drugs rather than the consequence of prolonged mismanagement of our food intake in this or even in previous generations – by us, our parents or our grandparents.

Then, having come to the conclusion that our body runs predominantly on sugar, retrospective logic is applied: namely some have come to think it was ever thus, and that we have always run on sugar as our main fuel. I myself look with atavistic eyes and so perceive things differently.

71

Unfortunately, this confusion has led astray even some of my fellow advocates of low carbohydrate nutrition. These enthusiasts have had some good results in practice, at least in the short term, by lowering carbohydrate. Yet they have clung to the new biology in terms of say, our supposed reliance on sugar from the last meal to keep energy going until the next, as well as to the idea of reliance on gluconeogenesis alone to see people through the night.

In other words, they have discarded the idea of our human body being historically suited to a diet consisting predominantly of the protein and fat from animal food, which went on supplying energy whether we ate or not for days at a time, and believe that the body is now dependent on sugar instead for its basic energy supply.

I love to theorise myself and admittedly do go astray, but the mistakes I am talking about are those that arise from our forgetting – or denying – our inheritance of many millions of years standing. One sees, for instance, very thin people trying to cut down on carbohydrates, who continue to cut down on 'evil' fat and who often abhor meat. To me, these people are in a state of semi-starvation and all because of misunderstood biology and the eagerly adopted but unproven theories that abound. Energy has to come from somewhere! And cutting down on both carbohydrate and fat is asking for trouble.

Relying mostly on protein for fuel, together with the sugar made from protein with the help of the adrenals, is also a way to great misfortune, as there is a limit to how much body protein can be spared in this way without harm. This process, say at night, also makes undue call on the catabolic (adrenal) hormones. Ironically, this same process happens with excess carbohydrate with little fat as well as with underfeeding.

Our origins as a distinct species being in the last Great Ice Age, our metabolism had to be both able to happily accept feast when it came, and also be prepared for occasional famine. In times of feast, for example after the capture of a large animal, there would be a great influx of nutrients to be either used or stored as fat for retrieval as needed in times of want.

Surely, if this was intended to be carbohydrate (and hence sugar), there would not be inbuilt restrictions as to how much sugar the bloodstream could carry safely at any one time? Surely, too, had nature intended carbohydrate to be our main fuel, our main food throughout the last Great Ice Age would have been carbohydrate foodstuffs, which of course was quite impossible as they were largely unavailable.

It is true that we need but little carbohydrate to satisfy our bodily requirements, however we must never forget how the design of our body is geared internally to run on fat as its primary fuel. Nor must we forget that, after a transition period and once the person is habitually on a low carbohydrate diet, the body gratefully reverts to more-or-less its original pattern of biology and so no longer runs on a constant emergency setting to cope with sugar overload.

One cannot overestimate the importance of efficiently providing both for energy as well as for the requisite building and repair materials for the body, not by mere calories, but by suitable nutrients in our food, particularly by fat and protein. Both are an essential part of the body's make-up, as I have said; fat is the more important energy provider but both the fat and the essential amino acids in protein are basic to health in that they provide the vital materials for tissue regeneration, including that of the arteries.

5 IN PRACTICE

My own medical work

Theorems come and go, and our detailed understanding of body processes gets ever more refined. Yet, as I have shown, our thinking about diet does not appear to become any less confused. One only has to go to the library, switch on the radio or open a newspaper to receive a plethora of conflicting advice. I think Prof. Glatzel was right when he said in his Introduction to the 5th edition of *Leben ohne Brot:*

> The value of a diet can only be judged on the basis of clinical experience and practical success and does not depend on biochemical or physiological explanations.
>
> (Glatzel 1975)

I feel that, ultimately, this has to be the case and I sincerely hope my own diet will be judged on its performance!

Low carbohydrate diets are slowly becoming fashionable and more is now written about them. I am thinking particularly of the so-called keto diets with minimal carbohydrate but also of my own more moderate level which does not need people to go into ketosis to be effective.

These minimal or restricted carbohydrate diets cannot, however, be applied indiscriminately to all patients, lest this brings such diets into disrepute the way that happened with cortisone because of its side-effects. Claims, for example, that all obese people will regain and retain their slender figure by merely reducing carbohydrate and doing lots of exercise are irresponsible: as I said before, things are not necessarily so straightforward, as I had found with my obese youngsters after puberty (Lutz 1964). Not only that, but a discredited diet may deprive people of the very real benefits this method can offer when done knowledgeably.

For a start, it is important that patients understand both any symptoms that may occur during the transition and the need to give their bodies enough time to adjust to a new way of eating. The transition to a low carbohydrate diet may well entail an increased intake of fat and protein. Many people have already passed a good proportion of their lives eating what amounts to an excess of carbohydrate and will have got into habitual ways of eating. Their bodies, too, will expect certain foods and will have made certain adjustments: this is because, over the decades, the body adapts and metabolic conditions may develop which are not to be changed overnight.

If people are already ill, it is important not only to get medical advice but to be monitored at intervals, especially during the transition. Here I must sound a note of extra caution against too sudden a transition. This is especially important in infarct-prone patients and for those in the so-called heart infarct age groups. Sudden change in itself can be both a challenge and a shock, sometimes with serious consequences. This is because sudden stress is apt to increase the tendency to coagulation and so to strokes and heart attacks. I remember saying as much to Robert Atkins years ago, when he first introduced his ultra-low carbohydrate diet.

In life, there are many sources of stress, especially for sensitive individuals, and I feel it is best not to add another one unnecessarily. I therefore advise anyone starting off on a low carbohydrate diet to take it SLOWLY and not to reduce carbohydrates TOO FAR or TOO FAST.

In my own practice – and remember I seldom find it necessary reduce carbohydrate further than to six or seven bread units – I would also urge certain patients not to increase fats too much and too quickly, especially at first. As regards this last point, this fat restriction would only be a temporary measure during the change-over period. In fact, with older patients, heart patients and those with arteriosclerosis, I may advise using both animal fat and vegetable oil for a time and especially at first. This applies particularly to patients who have an inherited tendency to thrombosis.

In the long term, it is important not to exclude or even to minimise fat intake. Indeed, for some people this means them making an extra effort to find ways of increasing their intake in a palatable way. After a time, this will no longer be an effort but become normal and even a delight, as they rediscover tasty dishes cooked with traditional fat using recipes from the days of their grandparents or before. When this happens, fat intake can be safely left to the patient's appetite.

What is interesting here is that I am not necessarily talking of a large amount of daily fat. (Please do not be misled by the description 'high-fat' diet!) Fat is so satiating that one does not necessarily need much of it, depending of course on occupation and energy expenditure. Once well-established on the diet, appetite for fat will regulate itself according to need.

For patients with existing arteriosclerosis it is important they eventually not only lower their carbohydrate intake to a daily maximum of six or seven bread units (72 – 84 g) but that they adhere to this amount in the long term. This is in order both to prevent any worsening of their condition and to give a chance for existing tissues damage to be repaired and their arteries to be regenerated as much as possible.

Over the years, I have used my own moderate diet with complaints as varied as gastric and intestinal maladies such as Crohn's disease and even ulcerative colitis, with blood level troubles, liver complaints and also many heart and circulatory problems, many of which respond very satisfactorily to this level of carbohydrate restriction.

On my diet, chronic conditions can, of course, take a time to show any real progress – often many months. I find that, done slowly and approached with caution, there is a gradual alleviation of symptoms, sometimes with the underlying condition or sensitivity remaining, as I found with my own arthritic hips. For instance, a sensitive intestine may stay liable to be irritated by certain foodstuffs but, if these are avoided in the long term, the patient may live pain-free and indeed symptom-free for years.

In my own case, my hips regained their mobility and I was able to live an active life for many years; later on, X-rays showed that the original deformation remained throughout. Ulcerative colitis was often slow to respond and could take years until full remission was gained: in the meantime, patients felt considerably better which encouraged them to persevere. With Crohn's disease, progress was much quicker.

Naturally, in both chronic and acute conditions, there may be relapses for a variety of reasons, one being not sticking closely enough to the prescribed diet. Even too many small deviations from it can hinder progress.

With acute conditions, once well-established on the diet, I found that many complaints responded to a low carbohydrate diet fairly quickly. Patients with angina pectoris, i.e. with impaired blood flow through the coronary arteries that supply blood to the heart, usually profit markedly from carbohydrate restriction and gain rapid relief. In fact, I do not remember having to send a patient for bypass surgery.

Moreover, I have the impression that fewer heart attacks occur on such a diet. From 29 of my patients who had lived for an average of 8.8 years on a low carbohydrate diet, only 5 of them (17%) suffered a further infarct, whereas according to the Framingham Study the prediction of a second attack would have been in the region of 35-50% (Lutz 1983).

In no way do I make a claim to cure cancer with my diet. However, I should mention that, after an operation say, for breast cancer, I have noticed that patients on my diet seem to recover particularly well and have shown little tendency to metastases. I am unable to say more than this, as I have not been able to give adequate follow-up to this observation.

In general, the rejuvenating effect of my modest diet has been very striking: it is interesting how many patients report improvements which are not directly related to the patient's presenting complaint: less anxiety, sounder sleep, more energy, happier digestion, better dental health, calmer nerves, improved muscle development and so on.

Nevertheless, it is important to realise that such a diet is no panacea, nor is it a quick fix to be used to get well and then to be discarded. Rather it is a way of looking at nourishment, a different way of choosing food and compiling meals. My diet is a way of eating for the long term: a diet for life, if you like, its composition suitable to promote health in the long term.

Hormonal balance

Once more back to my chickens! Those already familiar with my work may have noticed quite a few parallels between what

I observed in my chickens and what I was often observing in my patients. That these findings have direct relevance to human beings, I have in fact demonstrated through laboratory tests, hormonal investigations and the long-term monitoring of many patients.

Certainly, the background hormonal scenario had striking similarities. For with my patients, too, once the secretion of insulin was curtailed by a less provocative diet and the whole endocrine system came into a better and more harmonious balance, all manner of improvements in health came about and many of our diseases of civilisation responded favourably, including as I said, heart and circulatory diseases.

We saw that more carbohydrate given to Group VI hens was coupled with extra appetite for carbohydrate, presumably because of a rise in insulin in response, and that this was also linked to weight gain and increased arteriosclerotic change. Here I am reminded of my work with obese youth, who also had extra appetite for carbohydrate and who when tested were shown to have raised insulin levels.

What is interesting here are the striae which became evident on the skin of these youths. Now these skin lesions are essentially the same as the striae in arteriosclerosis, only that the latter are in the blood vessels not the skin. I was able to demonstrate clinically that these stripy 'stretch' marks were accompanied by heightened adrenal hormone secretion, of which they are a sign (Lutz 1964).

This hormonal activity is an expression of catabolic metabolism, that is the predominance of hormones which enhance the breakdown of tissue and hinder its build up. Glucocorticoid activity increases in response to stress and a lack of balance in the endocrine system is a stress.

Because of the hormonal seesaw – or balancing act – which exists between catabolism and anabolism, this catabolic predominance depresses the anabolic side, especially the growth hormone. Now, to stay healthy, the arteries particularly depend on a certain level of growth hormone, otherwise their resistance against various damaging influences and their regeneration potential decreases. And this because of an excess of carbohydrate in the diet!

Sadly, children already show the so-called milk spots, a beginning of arteriosclerosis, where lipids from the blood are integrated into the inner vessel walls. Tissue damage at these sites always precedes the lipid integration. Where the vessel wall is exposed to increased mechanical stress at the branch sites of the aorta, for example, the milk spots are more frequent as has been established experimentally by Prof. Hauss (19730 of Münster and Prof. Benditt (1977) of America. Both have pointed out many times that the primary factor is the tissue damage to which the body responds with repair measures, the integration of fats only secondary. This is the repair theory first propounded by Kaunitz that I mentioned in chapter 1, which I feel is not only highly plausible, but is supported by own work.

Not only is arteriosclerosis stress related but the risk factors for it are very interconnected, that is each is seen as being a risk factor for the other: obesity is a risk factor for diabetes, diabetes a risk factor for gout, gout and diabetes and obesity all risk factors for arteriosclerosis. These risk factors all seem to have issues of receptor defiance. Incidentally, the permeability of cell membranes is one of the cellular processes regulated by our endocrine hormones.

It follows that successfully treating any of the conditions that encourage arteriosclerosis, whether reducing stress, restoring normal weight, bringing down high blood pressure or reducing sugar, cholesterol or uric acid in the bloodstream should reduce the risk of arteriosclerosis developing.

As many of the risk factors potentiate each other, it is the more remarkable – and significant – that, in the majority of cases under my care, I have found that these conditions are amenable to treatment by the application of my modest diet.

Put simply, the common causal or predisposing factor for all the risk factors mentioned, is, in my view, carbohydrate excess; the main hope of preventing or alleviating any of these precursory conditions, is carbohydrate restriction. Many a time in my practice, I have monitored the fall of blood pressure, the stabilising of diabetes, the reduction of weight and much more.

With arteriosclerosis itself, when the disease is very advanced, I feel it may be too late to help other than by halting further degeneration. My views on this last point are not shared by two of my more radical low carbohydrate colleagues, both of whom claim to treat it by correcting the basic underlying imbalance which predisposed to the condition.

Whereas I saw the primary carbohydrate-induced imbalance as a disturbed hormonal system, Blake Donaldson, a heart specialist, who wrote the book *Strong Medicine,* saw it as a deficiency in essential amino acids, nutrients vital to the maintenance and repair of the arteries. As he says himself:

> . . . when hardening of the arteries sets in, as it does with all of us, the cells must be repaired. There is little in the food we take in that has the ability to grow cells except essential amino acids. These are readily available in fresh fat meat.
>
> Donaldson (1963)

In even advanced cases, Donaldson talks confidently of using corrective measures such as an early morning walk, plenty of red meat with the fat on three times a day and a demitasse of black coffee. He allows the occasional potato and perhaps a little fruit once weight has normalised.

Jan Kwasnieswki (1999), who wrote *Die Optimale Ernährung* (optimal nutrition) and whom I met in Poland, saw the basis for his treatment of arteriosclerosis as the rebalancing of the autonomic nervous system by eating food largely consisting of animal protein and fat, including plenty of eggs. These predisposing imbalances are of course not unconnected.

Perhaps having more courage than myself, both Donaldson and Kwasnieswki applied severe carbohydrate restriction to intermittent claudication and with apparent success. This was a type of arteriosclerosis of the legs and a disease which I was only hoping to prevent!

Was it then the hormonal system, the nervous system or the lack of amino acids that was the fundamental problem – or enzymes? When discussing the current epidemic of chronic degenerative diseases of the heart, arteries and nervous system in relation to the change from our ancient diet to the present day, Richard Mackarness, who has long been an advocate of a pre-cereal stone-age diet, put it this way:

When we suddenly confront our meat-adjusted body chemistry with high doses of refined starch, sugar and a host of new, synthetic chemicals, we invite a breakdown in our basic cell processes, of which we are already seeing evidence. It is difficult to realise just how enormously perilous it is to tamper with enzyme systems - the self-lubricating and self-repairing cogs of the body's physiological engine.

Mackarness (1963)

The regulation of specific enzyme systems is, by the way, one of the functions of the endocrine system.

Three of us with different viewpoints, all pointing to long-term imbalance in our intricately interwoven body systems! Not surprisingly, malfunction in one part can quickly lead to malfunction in another, whether between our hormonal regulators or other body systems. However, we all agree that, fundamentally, it is physiologically inappropriate diet that elicits this lack of harmony within the body.

I admit that it is sometimes necessary to use drugs to help individual patients with or without dieting. I am, however, reluctant to use pharmaceutical products to manipulate any of these imbalances without first having initiated a way of eating that does not continue to cause or recreate such imbalance. Better by diet than drugs!

In defence of fat, let me add a further quote of relevance from the same book by Mackarness :

> The primitive hunter in pursuit of food uses exactly the same nerve signal as the NASA scientist programming the computers which guide a landing on the moon. The difference is only in complexity. In both cases the work is done by the same sort of nervous system built of the same basic materials, chiefly animal fats. No nervous system has ever been built of starch or sugar, and to base a diet on carbohydrates, as millions do today, is to invite the problems of inadequately constructed and malfunctioning brain and nerves.
>
> Mackarness (1963)

Nor, for that matter, have any of our protein-laden arteries ever been built from starch or sugar!

And . . . ?

It is, I know, frowned upon to place too much weight on the value of animal experiments as a guide to human health – and mine was only a small study. Nevertheless, in the case of my chickens, I feel justified in allowing my trials to prompt many questions, so I now ask what else did the chickens share with us that is of interest?

Well, even within the same group, in terms of the amount of arteriosclerosis exhibited, not all chickens showed the same response to carbohydrate. Even given the same strain of hens, we saw that there was variation as to how many calories they chose to eat depending on the composition of their feed. This variety of response to stressors – for excess carbohydrate is a stressor – we find with people, too. Moreover, there are factors which can affect the development of arteriosclerosis that are neither mechanical, nor dietary, such as mental stress, viruses, lack of physical activity, environmental pollution and so on.

There will always be variations in response say, to the level of carbohydrate intake, so particular recommendations will not apply to everyone, hence my previous cautions. I find that, with my diet, once their symptoms have abated, people tend to find their own level of carbohydrate intake, a level at which they are comfortable, feel well and have no return of their symptoms. This can be lower or slightly higher than my general prescription of around six bread units.

I hesitate to say this next, as I am well aware of the sensitivity to some issues around diet held by some people. However, I must observe that the hens on a high amount of wheat grain, that is those on a feed consisting of almost half its weight as plant food, did badly both for arteriosclerosis and general health. Moreover, the wheat grain was not refined, but made from whole grain – which makes its own point.

Now, I have found with many gastrointestinal ailments, with my Crohn's patients for example, that it is precisely bread that is frequently badly tolerated, especially in any quantity. Indeed, much vegetable matter of any kind proved no more suitable for my gut patients than it did for the chickens. Vegetables are not the answer they are made out to be. They were marginal in early man's range of food and they certainly did not exist as bred nowadays for maximum sweetness. Myself, I scarcely touch them, but do allow the watery sort of salad vegetables to those who feel they need them or even root vegetables within the prescribed amount of carbohydrate.

A further problem with grain, which I have already touched on, was shared both by the chickens and many of my patients before they went on my diet. Remember that Group 1 hens ate less overall, including less calories. Put together well, that is with enough fat and protein, a low carbohydrate diet is very satisfying and so the appetite is self-limiting. But an excess of carbohydrate, as with Group VI, elicits a larger secretion of insulin, which stimulates the appetites and leads the hens back to the feed – or in our case to the breadbasket! If this goes on for some time, the weight rises, creating a risk factor for arteriosclerosis.

I also hesitate to use the word normalise, but shall I say there was a tendency in my chickens to grow healthy in the same way: fit muscles, sleek shape, good bone structure and fine plumage. In my patients, too, I saw this tendency to be more muscular, have better skin and better bones, to gain a better figure. There was also a tendency for body functions that were out of kilter to return to within acceptable parameters, for example stomach acid or blood values such as iron or calcium levels, triglycerides, uric acid or cholesterol.

A word about fat: those hens with a liberal allowance of fat – and mostly saturated fat – in their feed fared much better than those with a minimal allowance. I myself have found that a liberal amount of fat in my patients' diet gives substantial relief to those with gastro-intestinal troubles. I have been known to say that the gut cannot be cured without fat in the diet. And, of course, the satiating factor of fat does of course mitigate against over-eating in both people and hens.

As to the future, my successful chicken trials – for they were successful in showing that the lessening carbohydrate intake tended to lessen the incidence of arteriosclerosis – I feel point the way. That the main culprit was carbohydrate and not fat was clear. My own long experience with patients using a low carbohydrate diet, with free choice as to protein and fat, has fully confirmed the direction in which these trials point.

The way forward

That food should be fresh and as unspoilt as possible goes without saying. By unspoilt, I mean as little adulterated by chemicals as possible. I have always felt that to be so. I have likewise always encouraged health-promoting measures: I appreciate the value of clean air, fresh water and good farming methods and particularly the value of feeding cattle and sheep naturally.

We need to be wise and to be prudent. Excess never did any good. To my mind, in today's high carbohydrate world, to move forward, we also urgently need:

* to abandon the erroneous nutritional guidelines and to ridicule the fat theory: this in order to eliminate the advice to consume too little fat in favour of an unnatural and harmful preponderance of carbohydrate
* learn the lessons of our own history and the relevance of our origins that were not predominantly plant-based
* to stop demonising meat and instead to see it as an integral, health-giving part of our daily food
* encourage the reintroduction of traditional, beneficial fats, including animal fats, into our daily fare
* to understand that fat is our body's preferred primary fuel and that both protein and fat are vital constituents of body tissues and are building materials for repair
* to recognise that the eating of any more than a little carbohydrate constitutes a stress factor in itself
* to respect the body's self-protective mechanisms, lest we unwittingly do more harm: i.e. not think of receptor 'defects' but rather think of the shutting of the cell gates by the guards as a self-defence of last resort, e.g. to think of insulin resistance as laudable sugar resistance
* to remember that all warm-blooded animals have a limit to the amount of carbohydrate they can eat without upsetting their health – the point at which insulin has to prioritise too often the use of sugar as a fuel, which requires disadvantageous adjustments from our whole hormonal system
* to know that the average intake of carbohydrates in the western world already exceeds this limit
*conduct a large field study over many years, using people already following a low carbohydrate diet

As to this last, I myself tried for a great many years to get research projects instigated into the benefits of a low carbohydrate diet for various serious diseases. I remember going from university to university. Eventually I succeeded to get a trial done on Crohn's disease (Lorenz-Meyer 1996): the results clearly showed that reducing just sugar was not the answer, only when all carbohydrates were reduced was there a definite improvement.

I have long felt that the chapter on arteriosclerosis needs to be rewritten and that the current nutritional guidelines be revised in favour of less carbohydrate and more animal food. Given the size of our current population, our way of life and the current availability of various foodstuffs, we have to compromise on the menu. True, there is no way that say, the populations of London or Vienna could now survive by hunting but to advise that we avoid red meat and minimise animal fats is the height of physiological absurdity. My own advice to my patients: to sufficiently restrict carbohydrate and to eat as much protein – red or otherwise – and natural fat as their appetite dictates, would, I feel, offer far safer advice!

Finally, what of paramount importance do we learn about overall health from these trials that would most benefit arteriosclerosis? Even given individual variation, hormonally speaking I think that these trials point to a pressing need to reinstate a mutually beneficial relationship between the various endocrine hormones by abandoning an over-reliance on a species-inappropriate element in our food. I feel that I have shown that this cannot be adequately achieved except by sufficient daily restriction of carbohydrate. Give or take a little each way, I generally found about six bread units (72 g) to be the right amount to sustain this relationship satisfactorily.

In fact, in the light of my extensive clinical experience, backed up by the evidence of these chicken trials, my overall conclusion is that enough reduction in carbohydrate, regularly maintained, and with an adequate intake of protein and fat does indeed offer an invaluable therapeutic tool both for the prevention and treatment of many 'diseases of affluence'.

So yes, for the sake of arterial health, by all means fight against trans fats and commercial vegetable oils, yes by all means fight against denatured and chemically adulterated food, but remember, too, to fight against cholesterol-lowering margarines and low-fat products generally. Do encourage the gradual reintroduction of once familiar delights: let butter, suet, dripping and lard be once more used in flavourful cooking. Let meat be enjoyed with the fat on.

In other words, let us allow and enjoy those foods which will help to build robust bodies, strong arteries and healthy nervous systems and give a chance for people to know the peace of a stable and harmonious endocrine system.

Guten Appetit!

REFERENCES

ALLAN C B & LUTZ W (2000) *Life without Bread: How a Low-carbohydrate Diet can save your Life*
Keats, Los Angeles

ATKINS R C (1972) *Dr Atkins' Diet Revolution*
Bantam Books, N. Y.

BENDITT E P (1977) The Origin of Atherosclerosis
Scientific Am. 236 Nr 2, p.74

CLEAVE C L (1974) *The Saccharine Diseases*
John Wright & Sons, Bristol

DONALDSON B F (1963) *Strong Medicine*
Cassell & Co, London

ENIG M
Diet, Serum Cholesterol, and Coronary Heart Disease
in MANN (1993)

GLATZEL H (1974) 'Sinn und Unsinn in der Diätetik', VIII
Ischämie, Herzkrankheiten.
Med. Welt 25, 116

GLATZEL H (1982) *Wege und Irrwege moderner Ernãhrung*
Hippokrates Verlag, Stuttgart

GROVES B (2000) *Eat Fat, Get Thin*,
London: Vermillion

HAUSS W H (1973) Virchows Arch. Ges. Path. 359 p.135

KAUNITZ H (1976) 'Sind die Nahrungsfette bei der
Arteriosklerose von spezifischer Bedeutung?'
Munch. Med. Wschr. 119, 539.

KAUNITZ H (1978) Cholesterol & Repair Process in Arteriosclerosis
Lipids Vol.13, Nr.5, 373-374

KWASNIEWSKI J with CHYLINSKI M (1999)
Die optimale Ernährung,
Zuber, Vienna

LEWIN R (1988)
Bones of Contention,
Simon Schuster, New York

LORENZ-MEYER H, BAUER P, et al (1996)
Crohn's Study V
Scand. J. of Gastroenterology, 31, 778

LUTZ W (1964)
Das endocrine Syndrome des adipösen Jugenlichen
Wiener med. Wsch. 451

LUTZ W J, ANDRESEN G, BUDDECKE E (1969)
'Untersuchungen über den Einfluss einer kohlenhydratarmen
Langzeitdiät auf die Arteriosklerose des Huhnes'
Zsch. f. Ernährungswissenschaft 9, 222.

LUTZ W (1983)
Vortrag Kongress Deutsche Herzhilfe
Munich

LUTZ W (1986) *Dismantling a myth: the role of fat and carbohydrates in our diet*
Charles Thomas, Springfield, USA
and Selecta-Verlag, Munich

LUTZ W (1988)
Cholesterin und tierische Fette
SMV Edition Materia Medica, Munich

MACKARNESS R (1976)
*Not All in The Mind: How Unsuspected Food Allergy Can
Affect Your Body – And Your Mind*
Pan Books Ltd, London

MANN G V (1993)
Coronary Heart Disease: the dietary sense and nonsense
Janus Publishing Co., London

MANN G V (1977)
'Diet Heart, End of an Era'
New Engl. J. Med. 297.644.

McMICHAEL J (1977), 'Dietary Factors in Coronary Disease',
Eur J Cardiol 5, pp 447-52

OLSON R E (April 1980)
Toward Healthful Diets
Report to the US-Academy of Science, 28

OLIVER M (1983)
'Should we not forget about mass control of coronary risk
factors?'
Lancet II, 37

REAVEN G M (1976)
Commentary, Palo Alto Veterans Administration

RIDLEY M (1999), *Genome: The Autobiography of a Species
in 23 Chapters*, Fourth Estate

SALLMAN H., HARISCH G., SCHOLE J. (1976)
'Über den Einfluss einer kohlenhydratarmen Langzeitdiät auf
die Arteriosklerose des Huhnes'
Zbl.Vet.Med. A 23, 635-644

SCHOLE J, LUTZ W J (1988)
Regulationskrankheiten
F.Enke, Stuttgart

STEHBENS W
The pathology of Atherosclerosis
In MANN (1993)

STOUT R W & VALLANCE-OWEN (1969)
'Insulin and Atheroma'
The Lancet, May 31

WEITZEL G, BUDDECKE E I (1956)
Klin. Wschr. 34, 1171

YELLOWLEES W 1993)
A doctor in the wilderness
Janus Publishing Co., London, p 147

YUDKIN J (1971)
'Ernährung und Atherosklerose'
Medizin und Ernährung 12

Further details of the way of eating recommended by Dr Wolfgang Lutz can be found in my other books:

Uncle Wolfi's Secret: A Tribute to Dr Wolfgang Lutz
My Life Without Bread: Dr Lutz at 90

Made in the USA
Las Vegas, NV
19 March 2025